To harvey McCort
Class of 1961
Best wishes

— Lois Clendener
Nancy Yarn

75 YEARS BETWEEN THE PEACHTREES

A History Of

Crawford W. Long Memorial Hospital

Of Emory University

Lois Clendenen
with
Nancy Yarn

**SUSAN
HUNTER**

Atlanta, Georgia

Published by Susan Hunter Publishing, Atlanta, Georgia
Manufactured in the United States of America

54321

Publisher: Susan Hunter
Editor: Phyllis Mueller
Editorial Assistant: Nancy Kahnt
Book Design: Barbara Holcombe

Cover Photographs: Billy Howard

Library of Congress Cataloging-in-Publication Data

Clendenen, Lois, 1915-
    75 years between the peachtrees.

    Includes index.
    1. Emory University. Crawford W. Long Memorial
Hospital—History. I. Yarn, Nancy, 1899-
II. Title. III. Title: Seventy-five years between
the peachtrees.
RA982.A72E463 1987   362.1'1'09758231   87-31122
ISBN 0-932419-15-1

Pictured on back cover (L-R)
Lisa Yarn, Molly Greer, Glenice Johnson and Leroy Jackson.

CONTENTS

CHAPTER ONE
HOW IT ALL BEGAN 1

CHAPTER TWO
NAME CHANGES TO CRAWFORD W. LONG
    MEMORIAL HOSPITAL 23

CHAPTER THREE
NURSING EDUCATION 33

CHAPTER FOUR
DR. GLENN 51

CHAPTER FIVE
CRAWFORD LONG UNITS GO TO WAR 67

CHAPTER SIX
HOSPITAL EXPANSION 81

CHAPTER SEVEN
JESSE PARKER WILLIAMS STORY 89

CHAPTER EIGHT
IMPORTANT FIRSTS 95

CHAPTER NINE
CHAPEL PROGRAM 113

CHAPTER TEN
THE AUXILIARY TO THE CRAWFORD LONG
    HOSPITAL 121

CHAPTER ELEVEN
CARLYLE FRASER HEART CENTER 129

CHAPTER TWELVE
FURTHER EXPANSION 135

CHAPTER THIRTEEN
THE BUSINESS OF RUNNING A HOSPITAL 153

CHAPTER FOURTEEN
MEDICAL PERSONNEL STORIES 171

CHAPTER FIFTEEN
LONGTIME EMPLOYEE STORIES 187

CHAPTER SIXTEEN
THE MUSEUM 197

CHAPTER SEVENTEEN
SUMMING UP 203

ACKNOWLEDGEMENTS

Appreciation is extended to all who contributed to the contents of this book.

First, to Patsy Wiggins, coordinator of the Crawford W. Long Museum, who was ever patient, ready with suggestions and encouragement from the day the story moved from an idea to the time the manuscript was completed.

Next, to Mr. Render Davis, Assistant Administrator, who read the chapters as they came to him, in bits and pieces. Thanks to Pat Rogers and Eleanor Pascual for their accurate typing of copy that was pock-marked with additions, deletions, and corrections. Betty Jean Gates and Marjorie Winbush are remembered for the countless copies they made of the individual chapters and the final manuscript.

Mention must be made of Phyllis Mueller, editor at Susan Hunter Publishing, who carefully checked the manuscript page by page.

Thanks to all who gave interviews to Mrs. Nancy Yarn and me, and thanks for the help and anecdotes that reveal the "Crawford Long Spirit," and special thanks to Mr. Henry.

Finally, two people dear to me must be cited—John Clendenen, my patient and encouraging husband, and Anne Ludlow, retired Assistant Dean of the University College of the University of Rochester. Mrs. Ludlow has been my mentor since we shared bylines for a play we wrote in 7th grade. Her counsel then and now has been invaluable.

Lois Clendenen

DEDICATION

It is only in memory that we can turn back the pages of time that have become history.

75 Years Between The Peachtrees tells the story of Crawford Long Memorial Hospital.

This book is dedicated to all those who have ever had any part in founding, nurturing and maintaining the hospital's ultimate goal of healing performed with skill and compassion, concern and care for patients.

INTRODUCTION

This is the story of Crawford Long Hospital. Situated amid the gleaming towers of Atlanta's downtown business section, it combines the old with the new. How its service, its buildings, its staff, its good repute and its connection to Emory University came about is an exciting story that parallels Atlanta's growth.

What is termed the "Crawford Long Spirit" is an intangible, yet very present part of the whole hospital with its many clinics, offices and departments, miles of corridors, patient areas and waiting rooms, the Chapel and even the helipad, all dedicated to the well-being of the ill, impaired, and suffering. The dedicated staff keeps the hospital moving, to act, react, and interact.

Crawford Long Hospital has been fortunate in these who have served and are serving its patients presently. This history touches on their parts in Crawford Long's progress.

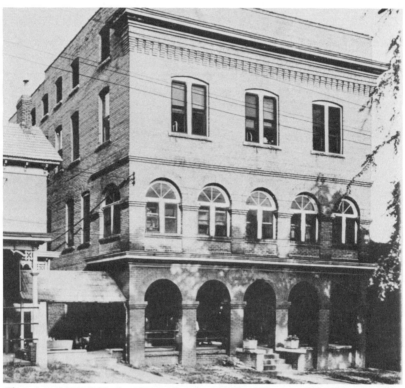

The original Davis-Fischer Sanatorium at 320 Crew Street, 1908-1909.

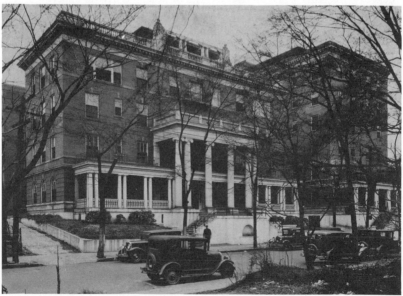

The original Davis-Fischer Sanatorium on Linden Avenue built 1910-1911.

CHAPTER ONE

HOW
IT ALL BEGAN

A hospital is more than a building. Just as a building is supported by its foundation, a hospital takes its philosophy from its founders. Crawford Long Hospital had as founders two people who believed that healing, not profit, was the basis for its being; concern for people was its motivating force. Dr. Edward Campbell Davis and Dr. Luther C. Fischer were physicians who turned dreams for a good hospital, affordable to middle class patients, into reality.

These two doctors from different backgrounds joined forces to open an office in the English-American Building at Broad and Peachtree Streets after Dr. Davis returned from duty in the Spanish-American War. For the benefit of the people of Atlanta, the two young doctors, drawn together by their love of people and devotion to medical progress, opened the doors of the Davis-Fischer Sanatorium on Crew Street on October 21, 1908. The hospital prospered.

Within the first year, bed capacity increased. By 1909, construction of a new hospital at 35 Linden Avenue became the nucleus for the present medical center.

DR. EDWARD CAMPBELL DAVIS

Dr. Davis, the elder of the successful physician team, met Dr. Fischer when he was Dr. Davis' pupil at the Atlanta College of Physicians and Surgeons. Their complementary association lasted until Dr. Davis died in 1931.

Dr. Davis was named Edward Campbell at his birth on October 11, 1867, to Eila Catherine Windler Davis and Dr. William Lewis

Gardner Davis in Albany, Georgia. His family called him Campbell. Accounts of his early life on a plantation tell of a happy childhood. Although his father died when Campbell was five years old, his mother managed her land and resources well, providing good educations for her eight children.

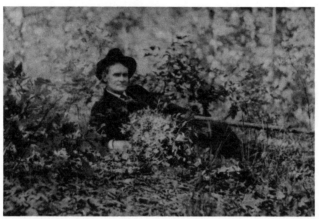

Dr. E. C. Davis in a moment of relaxation.

Campbell, whose uncle and elder brother W. L. were physicians, grew up in an atmosphere of medical conversation and lore. According to the account of Crawford Long History at its Fiftieth Anniversary, Dr. Shelley C. Davis (Campbell Davis' son) wrote, "Doctors of medicine from over the country, often guests in the Davis home, predicted a bright future for the two sons pursuing a career in medicine. It was understood the elder son would perpetuate his father's practice. With this background and association with leading physicians, broad avenues for the best surgical training of the times were open to him and he enthusiastically seized them."

After earning an A.B. degree from the University of Georgia in 1888, Campbell graduated in 1892 from the Medical School at the University of Louisville in Kentucky. He began practice in Atlanta with Dr. J. B. S. Holmes whose small infirmary was located on Cain Street directly behind the present Lane Bryant store. From then on, Campbell became known as Dr. E. C. Davis.

At that time, St. Joseph's Infirmary and Grady Hospital were the only Atlanta medical facilities with all school-trained doctors. Young doctors who were school-trained were impatient to use their knowledge and experience to try out their hard-earned skills.

It was during this exciting era that Dr. Davis met and courted the fair-haired Maria Carter, who became his wife and the mother of their eight children. During his service as major and chief surgeon in the Spanish-American War as a volunteer in the 2nd Georgia Volunteer Infantry they corresponded, and when he returned they married, in June 1899. Their first home was on Pine Street in downtown Atlanta.

Dr. Shelley Davis, writing of his father's feeling that a new hospital was needed, said, "The need for a new general hospital was so urgent Dr. Davis invited doctors with surgical training to his home and began a series of discussions that crystallized thinking into concrete planning.

"Dr. Bates Block and Dr. Michael Hoke were regular guests in Dr. Davis' home as was outstanding Baptist clergyman Dr. Len G. Broughton. They talked of nothing but a new hospital. Weeks grew into months before professional study finally produced practical plans to meet present and future needs for medical and surgical care for Atlanta's growing population.

"The very real problems of financing a hospital then presented further consideration and planning. At this time, the Hurt family had been making considerable civic and business contributions to the fast growing young city. Dr. C. D. Hurt was invited to join the doctor's planning sessions for suggestions on fund-raising."

During these latter meetings Dr. Fischer, son-in-law of Dr. Hurt, professed he, too, had dreamed of owning a hospital since he was a boy in Fayette County, Georgia.

When Drs. Block and Hoke cast their lot with Piedmont Hospital, and Georgia Baptists turned to building Georgia Baptist Hospital, Dr. Davis, anxious to have an independent hospital where patient welfare was the main consideration, withdrew from both groups. He joined Dr. Fischer who, although four years younger than Dr. Davis, had the business acumen of a more mature individual. It was their aim to build a third new hospital. And they did!

Their first venture soon outgrew its leased quarters in the old Railroad Hospital on Crew Street where the two young doctors started out with 18 beds for patients and faith in their venture, which included a fledgling nurse's training school of seven young women.

Dr. and Mrs. Davis lived for a short time in Dr. Holmes' Infirmary so he could be on call and keep living expenses down. Their first child, Shelley Carter Davis, was born there.

That Dr. Davis and Dr. Fischer were making their names known in Atlanta is evidenced by a Medical Association of Georgia program dated April 1907 naming Dr. Davis as the "5th District Councilor." Dr. Fischer was mentioned as a speaker on the subject "Should The Appendix Be Removed In All Cases Where The Abdominal Cavity Is Opened For Other Causes?" Both men published papers on some of their surgery cases.

When it became apparent the hospital on Crew Street was inadequate, a search was started for a new locale.

Mrs. Shelley Davis, widow of Dr. Shelley Davis, Sr., delights in relating this family story told to her by her mother-in-law. Maria Davis was awaiting the birth of her fifth child. Following the custom of the day to hide visible signs of pregnancy, she donned her "great cape to take her evening constitutional" as prescribed by her doctor. Her late evening walk took her past the Morris Brandon property on Linden Avenue. Each night she told her husband of what a fine location it would be for his new hospital.

Finally, she persuaded him to have a look at it. He was impressed, and so was Dr. Fischer, although people were skeptical of a location "in a place so far out of town." These gloomy predictions were brushed aside, the property was purchased, and plans for building the 85-bed Davis-Fischer Sanatorium were begun.

Horror over the loss of life in a fire that burned down a wooden hospital in Montreal, Canada, where 12 people died, caused a change of plans. Dr. Shelley Davis tells this story, "Immediately Dr. Fischer, treasurer of the Davis-Fischer partnership, began figuring to find means for changing their building plans to a completely fireproof building. The high cost of the modern fireproof construction exceeded personal funds and even frightened possible donors to the new hospital."

The two doctors decided to incorporate. On May 15, 1910, Judge J.D. Pendleton signed the papers that made Dr. E. C. Davis and Dr. L. C. Fischer equal stock holders with shares of $2,500 apiece.

"Then," goes on the 1948 history, "It happened at this time Dr. Davis operated on Captain Robert Lowry, then president of the Lowry National Bank. The grateful patient agreed to loan the additional needed funds. The new hospital building was assured." The Davis-Fischer Sanatorium opened its doors in 1911.

From an account of the life of Dr. Davis by Isabella Arnold Bunce, that appeared in the July 1950 issue of the Journal of the

Medical Association of Georgia, comes praise for the surgical skill of Dr. Davis. She wrote, "Dr. E. C. Davis always kept pace with the progress of his profession. He bought and installed the first freezing microtome. With this, fresh tissue sections could immediately be prepared and diagnosed on all cases of suspected cancer to determine the extent of surgery needed while the patient was still on the table.

"His greatest feats were accomplished by his skill and originality in gynecologic and abdominal surgery."

Dr. Davis was always prompt in the operating room. He began his surgery at or before 8 o'clock each morning. In addition, he would have numerous emergencies carried in day or night from a radius of three hundred miles or more.

"During the day, Dr. Davis would take time out only for a short lunch. He was constantly surrounded by doctors, interns and nurses as he made his rounds where he frequently had twenty or more patients in the hospital.

"Besides being one of the South's most distinguished surgeons, he was one of the best loved of his time. To the young doctors, he meant as much as their surgical hero but a friend as well."

A firm believer in antiseptic technique, Dr. Davis is remembered as a pioneer in the use of rubber operating room gloves that many of his contemporaries found cumbersome, blunting the sensitivity of their fingers in complicated surgery.

It was said of him, "Dr. Davis was almost uncanny in recognizing the signs of eclampsia and other toxemias of pregnancy. The expectant mothers were given constant care with examinations and regular laboratory checks."

As time passed, the Davis-Fischer Sanatorium prospered, and the debt to Captain Lowry was repaid. There were hard times, too. In the 1915 minutes of the annual stockholder's meeting, it was recorded: "The year from March 1, 1914 to March 1, 1915 has been financially the hardest year that we, certainly in this generation, have ever seen." As the hospital's reputation grew, things improved.

In 1917, negotiations were made to purchase an adjoining lot to build a new building. It is said that about this time, the doctors, by use of persuasion, were able to get smooth paving on Linden Avenue to replace the worn, uneven cobble stones.

In 1914, Dr. Davis went to London to represent the American Medical Association at the World Medical Congress. While there, he studied methods and equipment of hospitals and he ordered new surgical instruments for his hospital back home.

While Dr. Davis was still in London, the first World War broke out in Europe. Dr. Davis returned home as a steerage passenger, and his new equipment came three months later. In April 1917, President Woodrow Wilson declared the United States at war with Germany and her allies.

Again we return to Dr. Shelley Davis' history for a first hand account of that wartime crisis. He wrote: "As America was drawn into the war so were its doctors and nurses. Medical schools were asked to organize medical units and Dr. Davis, having continually served as a professor at Emory University and having maintained a military rank also, was asked to organize Atlanta doctors for service.

"Country came before self, home, family, or the Sanatorium. Such outstanding medical men as Dr. Edgar H. Greene, Dr. Frank Boland, Sr., Dr. C. W. Strickler, Sr., Dr. Charles Dowman, Sr., Dr. Allen H. Bunce, Dr. Jake Sauls, Dr. John Fitts, Dr. Edgar G. Ballenger, Dr. Charles E. Lawrence, Dr. F. M. Barfield and Dr. Murdock Equen rose to the call and became part of Atlanta's Emory Unit for war service.

"Thirty-five physicians, one hundred and fifty-three enlisted men, and one hundred registered nurses finally reported at Davis-Fischer Sanatorium in March, 1918 to be transported to nearby Camp Gordon for overseas preparation.

"Although Dr. Davis remained president of the Sanatorium, Dr. Fischer was left to manage the hospital from March, 1918 until the Armistice in November of that same year."

Because of his work in France, Dr. Davis was recognized by General John J. Pershing and was decorated by King Alexander of Greece.

Dr. Davis, wearing the rank of a lieutenant colonel, returned to the Davis-Fischer Sanatorium just in time to join the war on influenza that was then raging in epidemic force all across the nation. Public buildings were closed and hospitals, including Davis-Fischer, overflowed with patients. In August of 1921, a new building opened, with a bed capacity of 150.

Dr. Davis was the devoted father of lively children named Shelley, Catherine, Page, E. C., Jr., Ria, Robert Carter, Sarah, and Teddy. Life in the Davis home during these years was pleasant and family-oriented. Dr. Davis and his family enjoyed riding their horses "Faith," "Hope," and "Charity."

Friends were always welcome at their home: its hospitable doors were opened to a couple who asked for a few nights' lodging while they searched for a dwelling. Dr. Davis referred them to Mrs. Davis for her consent. She gave it and they stayed for five years.

There were family vacations at Pass-a-Grille Island, Florida where Dr. Davis enjoyed fishing for tarpon and free time with his family. Every July, for many years after WWI, Dr. and Mrs. Davis entertained the Emory Unit #43 people and their friends with a barbecue at the Davis Farm on Northside Drive.

Honors came to him in many forms.

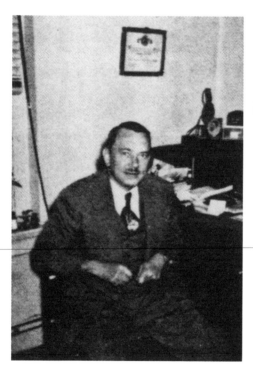

Dr. Shelley Davis

He was chosen president of the Fulton County Medical Society in 1925 and served as president of the Medical Association of Georgia from 1910-11, and became an early Fellow of the American College of Surgeons. He was awarded an honorary Doctor of Laws degree by Emory University in 1930, recognizing his services as "Daddy" of the WWI Emory Unit #43 and for his leadership in the advancement of the medical education in the South.

Base Hospital #43 presented a portrait of their former commander in his uniform to be hung in the Emory Hall of Fame.

He was Chairman of the Board of Trustees of the Fulton County Medical Society at the time of his death, and was Professor Emeritus of Gynecology at the Emory Medical School.

An article in the "Journal of the Medical Association of Georgia," published in March 1939, lauded Dr. Davis' memory, saying: "He was an outstanding medical practitioner." Dr. J. Calvin Weaver once said, "Dr. Davis could be compared to St. Luke, the Beloved Physician."

He retired from active medical practice in 1929 when his health, never robust since his duty in France in 1918, failed. As his vision dimmed, Mrs. Davis was ever at his side to help him move easily around the familiar rooms of their home. In praise of her, he said, "In a great measure, any achievements credited to me came because of my wife."

He died on March 11, 1931. He was laid to rest in West View Cemetery with full military honors.

Dr. Davis' funeral service was conducted by Dr. Richard O. Flinn and the Reverend E. A. Fuller at the First Baptist Church. He was warmly remembered for his service as a major and surgeon of the Spanish-American War and as the commanding officer of the Base Hospital at Blois, France during World War I.

"He was a surgeon of outstanding skill who won an enviable reputation in his profession and to those outside it, he was known as a man of unusual charm," were the words of tribute paid to his memory.

Pall bearers were Dr. L. C. Fischer, Dr. J. C. Ivey, Dr. E. H. Greene, Mr. H. Tanner, Mr. W. S. Spalding and Mr. N. D. Malcolm. The honorary escort was made up of Fulton County Medical Society members and friends from the Base Hospital #43 and the Medical Corps Unit. Also present to pay their respects were workers from the Davis-Fischer Sanatorium.

To his wife and family, he left "the sweetest memory ever treasured." To Crawford Long, he left two dedicated physicians—his two sons—Dr. Shelley C. Davis and Dr. Robert Carter Davis, both Crawford Long doctors; and two grandsons. Dr. Robert Carter Davis, Jr. is at Crawford Long and Dr. Shelley Carter Davis is at Emory Hospital. Render S. Davis, another grandson, serves as Assistant Administrator at Crawford Long.

This third-generation Davis physician learned the name "Davis" made a lasting impression on one patient. He said, "I was asked to see her, went by and introduced myself. She was lying in bed, just as cute as she could be. The minute I said, 'Davis,' she reached out and held my hand as she said, 'Well, now I'm going to be okay.' I was confused until she said, 'Are you any kin to Dr. E. C. Davis? He was my doctor and Dr. Shelley Davis took care of me after Dr. E. C. died. After Dr. Shelley died, your daddy took care of me. You know I'm ninety years of age. Now you're my doctor. I've never had a doctor whose name wasn't Davis.' "

"I teased her," said Dr. Shelly Davis, "and told her that every doctor named Davis who took care of her had died."

Dr. E. C. Davis was decorated by General John Pershing for his service in World War I.

Mrs. Shelley Davis, Sr. widow of Dr. E. C. Davis' son, Dr. Shelley Davis, still has the citation which says "U.S. Army Citation to Lt-Col.Edward C. Davis, M.D., for exceptional meritorious and conspicuous services at Base Hospital, Number 43, France, American Expeditionary Forces.

"In Testimony thereof, and as an expression of appreciation of these services I award him this citation awarded April 19, 1919"

—John J. Pershing
Commander-In Chief

Dr. Davis is still remembered by a former patient, Agnes Roberts, who celebrated her eighty-fifth birthday in 1986.

She remembers, "I was run over by a car at Piedmont and Ivy Roads. When my arm turned black, my mother decided to call Dr. E. C. Davis. He came right out and took me to the Davis-Fischer Sanatorium in his car. He was a grand man. He took me to the x-ray and then put a plate in my arm. He told me he did that for wounded soldiers in France during the war. He said the plate was temporary. That arm healed up and the plate stayed in place for twenty years and then it had to come out. Dr. Davis was a wonderful man."

DR. LUTHER C. FISCHER

Luther Fischer was born on a farm near Senoia in Fayette County on August 15, 1873. Later, in the custom of the times, he added the middle initial 'C' to give his name balance and dignity.

In 1899, he added an M.D. to the end of it. When Dr. Luther C. Fischer died in 1953, he was known as co-founder of Crawford

Long Memorial Hospital and for his philanthropy.

After Fischer's death, Boisfeuillet Jones, assistant secretary of the Emory Board of Trustees, sent Mrs. Fischer a copy of a memorial service that was read and made part of the Board's permanent record at its annual meeting on October 27, 1958.

The memorial reviewed Dr. Fischer's life and his devotion to the growth of Crawford Long Hospital, closing with: "Dr. Fischer's large benefactions for the good of mankind during his life and by his final bequests will serve as a perpetual memorial to this successful, energetic and generous citizen who has been one of our section's outstanding philanthropists. Generations yet unborn will call him blessed."

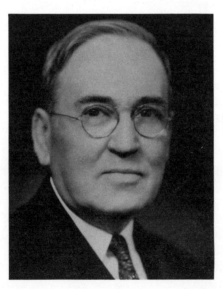

Dr. Luther C. Fischer

George W. Woodruff and C. H. Candler, Jr. had praise "for the great good Dr. Fischer did for the people of the community in founding, then giving to charity Crawford Long Hospital."

Goodrich C. White, president of Emory University, in a personal letter to Mrs. Fischer wrote in part: "His generous contribution to the ongoing and future of Emory University will, of course, be a permanent part of Emory's history."

Young Luther Fischer, son of Sally Rainey Fischer and Hartford Fischer, often told of his early ambition to be a physician skilled in healing people of all classes and to own a hospital.

His father wanted Luther to be a lawyer, but his mother, who had noted her son's sensitive hands at work with animals, encouraged him to keep alive his goal of studying medicine.

He went to college in New York and came back to Georgia to attend the Atlanta College of Physicians and Surgeons (now Emory School of Medicine). To earn his tuition, he worked for The Coca-Cola Company, a new business in Atlanta. He learned about business as he traveled from state to state selling Coca-Cola syrup. He graduated with an M.D. degree in 1899, took postgraduate work in New York City, and later in Vienna, and Berlin.

Upon his return to Atlanta, he became a member of the faculty of the Atlanta College of Physicians and Surgeons as professor of anatomy and clinical surgery. He also entered the office of Dr. C. D. Hurt, his future father-in-law.

He and "Miss Lucy" were married in 1900. They had no children.

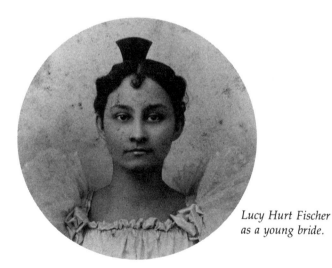

Lucy Hurt Fischer as a young bride.

Dr. Fischer left his father-in-law's office to work with Dr. Davis and open the Davis-Fischer Sanatorium in 1908. Dr. Fischer's own words of this venture, written in 1937, are preserved in Franklin Garrett's *Atlanta and Environs, Vol. II.*

He wrote: "It was in 1908 that the late Dr. E. C. Davis and I saw the great necessity of a private hospital as there existed in Atlanta at that time only St. Joseph's Infirmary and Grady Hospital and some other small private institutions . . .

"There being a great need for hospitals for private patients, and both of us having the ambition, it was necessary for us to build and operate an institution of our own. Dr. Stockhard had, with some associates, built a small hospital on Crew Street. In his day, it was operated as a private hospital mostly for medical cases with a limited capacity of about 18 beds.

"In 1908 Dr. Stockhard decided to discontinue the operation of his hospital, so Dr. Davis and I leased the building for a term of two years with the privilege of renewal, and we opened the Davis-Fischer Sanatorium. An apartment house across the street was leased for the nurses' living quarters. This gave a total bed capacity for twenty-six patients."

Dr. Fischer performed the first operation in the new building on February 27, 1911. He kept a little jar containing the 26 small polished pebbles he removed from the gall bladder of a patient that day as a conversation piece. He liked to point them out and laugh as he said, "Those are from my first operation in the new hospital, and the patient is alive and well today."

After the loan from Captain Lowry was paid, expansion continued. In August of 1921, a new seven-story building was completed, bringing the bed capacity up to a hundred and fifty.

As time passed, against pessimistic advice that a five-story nurses' home to be built on West Peachtree Street would be too big, Dr. Fischer pushed for a seven-story structure. As usual, his optimism won out.

Later, three apartment houses on Prescott and West Peachtree Streets were purchased and remodeled for the use of nurses and interns. Still later, the Byron Apartment Hotel at the foot of Linden Avenue on West Peachtree was purchased as quarters for interns and their families.

As the nurses' home neared completion in the early 1940s, Dr.Fischer started construction on a maternity center. One does not have to travel far in Atlanta to find children, their mothers and grandmothers who were safely born at Crawford Long. When the Emily Winship Woodruff Maternity Center, with all the latest scientific equipment, was dedicated on January 17, 1942, Dr. Fischer said, "This center is dedicated to medical science in the fight it is waging to lower mortality rates among mothers. Statistics show that 16,000 women lost their lives in childbirth last year. By means of medical examination, pre-natal care and the education of expectant mothers, this high mortality rate can be materially lowered, and it is the purpose of this center to dispense such vital services to those women who otherwise might not be able to obtain them."

Lectures on prenatal care, preparation of food, diet and the making of infant and mother apparel were started. A fee of $1 was charged to provide routine laboratory examinations. Alice Thompson was named the center's director.

The architect for the first and second buildings was E. C. Wachendorff, son of a pioneer Atlanta family. The contractor was E. P. Hefner; concrete work was done under the direction of H. W. Beers and Charles Loridans of the Southern Ferro-Concrete Company. Maternity Center Building architects were Hentz, Adler and Shutze. The contractor was the Barge Thompson Co. under the direction of W. B. Thompson.

The nurses' home architects were Hentz, Adler and Shutze with Hal Hentz directing and Warren Armistead as associate. The contractor was the Beers Construction Co.

During these hospital expansion years Dr. Fischer had other interests that proved to be serendipitous for the hospital. His farm, "Flowerland" where he raised fine stock and established a beautiful garden, was opened for the enjoyment of the public. Meat, eggs, poultry, milk, fresh vegetables, and watermelons were sold to the hospital to provide patients with nutritious, taste-tempting meals. Flowerland's watermelons became an everyday in-season treat for staff and patients for many years.

Dr. Fischer and the local 4-H Club admire his prize-winning cattle.

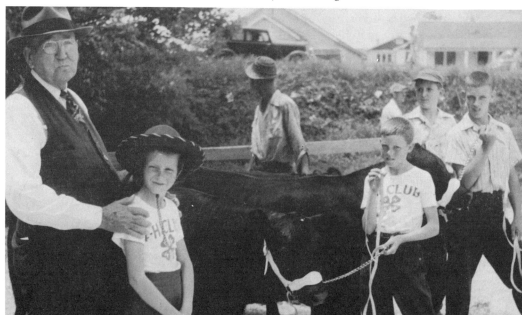

Melissa Jack Hurt remembers "Uncle Luther" and his wife Lucy.

She said, "Both Uncle Luther and Crawford Long Hospital loomed large in our lives and background through the years. On December 12, 1900, Luther C. Fischer married Lucy Hurt, sixth child of Dr. Charles Hurt. She was named for her grandmother, Lucy Apperson Long Hurt. This grandmother was a relative of Dr. Crawford Long."

Dr. Charles Hurt, Lucy's father, studied medicine in Atlanta and Augusta and practiced medicine in Huntsboro until 1884. He moved to Columbus, Georgia where he was president of the Board of Health and a member of the School Board and chairman of the Board of Stewards at St. Luke's Methodist Church.

In 1893, at the suggestion of his brother, Joel Hurt, the Charles Hurt family moved to Atlanta and Dr. Hurt took the position as physician for the Atlanta and Edgewood Street Railway Company.

The Hurt family lived in Inman Park in a house Dr. Hurt had built. It was during this time he became associated in practice with Dr. Fischer.

When Melissa Jack married Charles Davis Hurt, III in 1933, she "became a part of the family circle around Uncle Luther and Aunt Lucy.

"I remember," she said, "their hospitable home, Flowerland, and their gracious sharing of it with the large family connection. They gave receptions for brides like me coming into the family, wedding receptions for those moving out of town, and I recall the famous Sunday afternoon Open House. At these, an exuberant Uncle Luther marched us through the gardens telling the stories of all the flowers. Gentle, quiet Aunt Lucy remained in the house smiling over everyone. Childless, they enjoyed surrounding themselves with their large family connection.

"And I remember so vividly the commanding figure of Uncle Luther at Crawford Long Hospital, his office, his stories, his air of presiding over us and always taking time with us. All of us were proud of Uncle Luther and proud to be patients in his hospital."

A newspaper account tells of an earlier gift of a charity ward Dr. Fischer had given to the hospital in memory of his mother and her encouragement to him. This was a part of the Annex when it opened.

In this ward, furnished with the most modern fixtures, beds

were set aside for worthy charity cases of any staff member. A newspaper clipping dated 1921 mentions Davis-Fischer as one of the few private hospitals to provide a charity ward.

When Dr. Davis died on March 11, 1931, Dr. Fischer became president of the hospital. Three weeks later the name was changed to the Crawford W. Long Memorial Hospital.

Over the next few years many changes took place under the eye of Dr. Fischer. He was the prime mover in bringing Georgia into the United Hospital Service Association.

He was responsible for the removal of the word "illegitimate" from birth certificates in Georgia.

As a staunch promoter of group hospitalization insurance, Dr. Fischer spoke to civic and other groups of its success elsewhere. He emphasized the benefit of the plan to less fortunate families who, with it, would be relieved of worry over huge hospital bills.

He was one of seven hospital petitioners for the new law. The others were Dr. P. H. Oppenheimer (Emory Hospital), Thomas H. Hancock (Atlanta Hospital), W. D. Barker (Georgia Baptist Hospital), George R. Burt (Piedmont Hospital), Jessie M. Candlish (Egleston Memorial Hospital) and Estes Doremus (St. Joseph Infirmary).

On March 30, 1937, Governor E. D. Rivers, a recent Crawford Long patient, under the sculptured gaze of Dr. Crawford Long's statue at the hospital, signed the new group hospitalization bill as Dr. Fischer and Rep. E. L. Almada of Walton County looked on.

With the governor's signature the law was sealed to place hospital services within the reach of all, rich and poor alike.

In early 1937, Dr. Fischer's beloved "Miss Lucy" died. In the fall of 1938 Dr. Fischer and Alice Thompson, hospital Superintendent of Nurses, were married in a quiet ceremony in the study of the Rev. Richard Orme at the North Ave. Presbyterian Church in the presence of a small circle of friends. After a honeymoon spent in New York City they returned to Flowerland.

On December 11, 1938, Dr. Fischer announced that he had given Crawford Long Hospital back to the people of Atlanta in the form of a trust under the direction of a group of men he felt would carry out his well-known "concern for the man of modest means." The transfer was made without reservation or restriction.

At that time Harold Martin, a respected Atlanta writer, quoted Dr. Fischer as saying, "I dream of this hospital as a place of healing for the man of modest means who won't accept charity. To my mind, such an institution is the greatest need of Atlanta today.

"This is the sort of place I visualize for Crawford Long. I think I have found the men who can make that dream come true.

"They are Ernest Woodruff and his son George; Guy Woolford; T. K. Glenn; A. A. Acklin; Armand May; J. D. Robinson; Dr. Frank Boland, Sr.; J. N. Reisman; Dr. Wadley Glenn and J. E. Sanford."

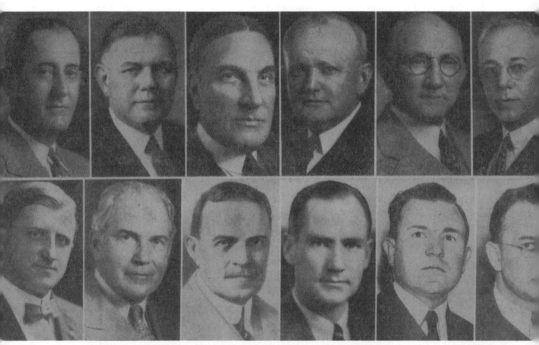

Members of the new board of directors which would administer Crawford Long. Top row, left to right, A. A. Acklin, T. Guy Woolford, James D. Robinson, J. E. Sanford, Thomas K. Glenn, J. N. Reisman. Lower row, Dr. Frank K. Boland, Armand May, Ernest W. Woodruff, Dr. Wadley Glenn, George Woodruff, Russell C. Nye. Mr. Nye was not a member of the board, but was being trained by Dr. Fischer to carry on executive duties in years to come. (Photo from the Atlanta Journal/Constitution)

(Later, Dr. Joseph H. Boland and Wilbur Glenn became board members.)

"It's all theirs now. The two buildings here on Linden St., 225 beds in all, and a lot across the street where I hope someday to see a third building rise.

"Seven years ago, looking to this time, with full agreement before he died of my good friend and associate Dr. E. C. Davis, the charter of Davis-Fischer which we built was changed to operate as an eleemosynary institution without profit.

"The name was changed to Crawford W. Long Memorial Hospital in tribute to that great Georgian, the discoverer of sulphu-ric ether for anesthesia.

"Then I kept the title to the property, but today I turn it all over to the trustees I have named. It is theirs to run and all I ask is the same job to do that I've been doing all along. When the time comes I'm too tired to work any more, I can go home to Flowerland and watch the roses bloom, content that the job is in good hands."

Dr. Fischer gave Flowerland and his 138-acre estate in Chamblee to the same board of trustees at that time.

As president of the new board, Dr. Fischer continued his personal attention to administrative affairs of the hospital. Dr. Glenn, also a member of the boards of Grady and Emory Hospitals, was named secretary.

Dr. Carl C. Aven, president of the Fulton County Medical Society, joined Dr. Edward H. Greene, president-elect of that organization, and Dr. J. L. Campbell, chairman of the Georgia Medi-cal Association, in praise of Dr. Fischer's gift. Dr. Greene said at that time, "In giving of Crawford Long Hospital to a board of trustees, Dr. Fischer has done a magnanimous act."

He commanded a staff of 200 of Atlanta's best physicians, nurses and hospital workers in the institution whose affiliation with the United Hospitals Service Association provided a way for pa-tients to make repayments for hospitalizations. On January 21, 1940, Dr. Fischer announced the transfer of Crawford Long Hospital, now valued at $1 million, to Emory University.

At the same time the board told of the purchase of adjoining property as a site for a new $300,000 Nurses' Home and a Maternity Center. The Nurses' Home, with Hal Hentz as architect, would be on the Hoke Smith property on West Peachtree St. It would accom-modate 96 student nurses.

Dr. P. H. Oppenheimer, dean of the Emory University School

of Medicine, accepted the deed saying in part, "It is believed that this hospital will become an important unit in the Medical Center development and, in accordance with the ideals of its founders, will render a great service to the community. Emory welcomes the cooperation of the Crawford Long Memorial Hospital organization and in turn will give its best cooperation to their work."

A portrait of Dr. Fischer, unveiled in the auditorium of the Nurses' Home on November 27, 1949, was presented by the staff doctors, nurses and hospital employees. Painted by Benedict Milner, it now hangs in the hospital lobby.

The portrait committee members were Dr. Frank Boland, chairman; Drs. E. H. Green, W. W. Daniel, Wadley Glenn, McClaren Johnson, M. P. Pentecost and Mrs. Macie Stephens, director of service coordination.

The portrait was a tangible sign of the respect of Dr. Fischer's co-workers; it was a time to remember some of his accomplishments.

Remembered was the World War II shortage of metals for civilian use that delayed the move of the operating room from the fourth floor of the "A" Building. An $800 piece of equipment was needed to get the air conditioning going. But the head of the War Production Department refused to give permission to meet this need. Dr. Fischer wrote a persuasive letter to Eleanor Roosevelt. Permission was granted.

In his regular Christmas greeting to each employee in 1942, he included a war stamp as a token of appreciation for their cooperation in the war effort.

That Dr. Fischer had a soft side as well-known as his medical skill and his business acumen is preserved in a fat scrapbook on file in the Museum.

Here are found sentimental and uplifting poems and positive attitude articles of philosophy along with pictures of friends, babies, his beloved Flowerland and photos of his prize-winning stock animals.

There are clippings of favorite columnists, personal greetings and letters of appreciation for his gifts of roses.

Of scientific interest, there are published papers of medical operation procedures as performed by Dr. Fischer.

To further studies and research among young physicians of the Fulton County Medical Society, Dr. Fischer offered monetary prizes for original essays.

In 1925, Dr. Davis announced that Dr. Fischer would award

two prizes of $100 each, a large sum of money back then.

Winners were Dr. M. H. Roberts for his paper on "Physical Pigmentation of the Newborn", and Dr. R. H. Wood and G. A. Williams for their study on "Primitive Human Hearts".

The 1926 winner was Dr. D. C. Elkin for his paper "Intra-plural Pressure in Post Operative Atcleclasis". Judges were Dr. E. C. Davis, E. B. Black and A. H. Bunce.

One letter still preserved says: "Dear Dr. Fischer, It was indeed a happy surprise to me to be selected to receive one of the Fischer Awards for medical research during the year 1936. Winning the award means much to me not only because of the prize itself but because of the stimulus it will give me to strive for bigger and better things in the future. I wish to take this opportunity of thanking you for the award and for the gorgeous flowers presented me at the banquet—Sincerely yours, Lola Denmark."

His reply to her was:

Dear Dr. Denmark,

Thank you so much for your letter of January 11. It was a pleasure and privilege for me to offer the award through the Fulton County Medical Society for good work. Am so delighted that you were a winner.

I am more than repaid to feel that a group of doctors, especially the younger ones are getting inspiration from this.

With kindest regards and best wishes I am

Very truly yours,
L. C. Fischer

Excerpts from a 1937 hand-written letter from Dr. Amey Chappel expresses a similar gratitude for an award presented to her by Dr. Fischer for a paper she wrote: "Anemia and Pregnancy, A Three Year Study on Negro Women."

Dr. Chappel wrote: " . . . Combined with the pleasure which I am experiencing in sharing one of the Fischer Awards is a sense of humility . . . Dr. Bivens and I divided the check equally. Part of mine will be spent for some medical books which I have wanted and could not afford. The balance will be spent probably on more research . . . If anything was needed to complete the pleasure of Thursday evening it was provided by the box of lovely red roses . . ."

Two letters from Dorothy Walker, a 6th grade school teacher, report the progress of youngsters he was interested in—children of his farmworkers and others. Letters from local ministers show appreciation for help he had given to them for their needy or worthy church members.

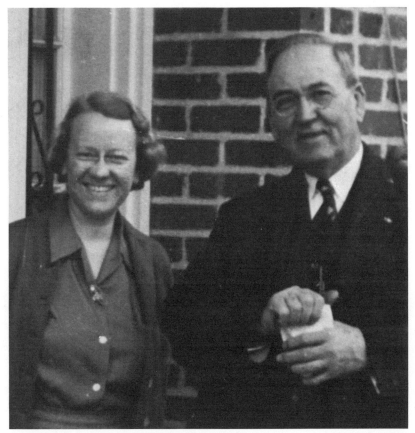

Alice Thompson Fischer and Dr. Fischer.

An appealing account of letter exchanges between Dr. Fischer and a humble man tells of his reply "thank you" letter to the man who had expressed gratitude for a check sent him for his wife's operation expense. A second note tells that not only did the woman recover, she had two more children after age forty. When she later returned to Crawford Long for further surgery, she gave Dr. Fischer and fervent prayer credit for her recovery. She died in 1972 at age 91.

When Dr. Fischer died in his eighty-second year, the bulk of his estate was left to care for indigent patients.

Crawford Long Hospital, now accredited by the Joint Commission on Accreditation of Hospitals, is a member of the American Hospital Association, the Georgia Hospital Association and the Council of Teaching Hospitals of the Association of American Medical Colleges.

In addition to a diploma School of Nursing, Crawford Long also trains health professionals in medical and radiologic technology. Its training program of interns and residents is part of the Affiliated Hospital Residency Program of Emory University School of Medicine.

Crawford Long Hospital is a viable tribute to Dr. Davis and Dr. Fischer, and bears the name of Georgia's most famous pioneer doctor.

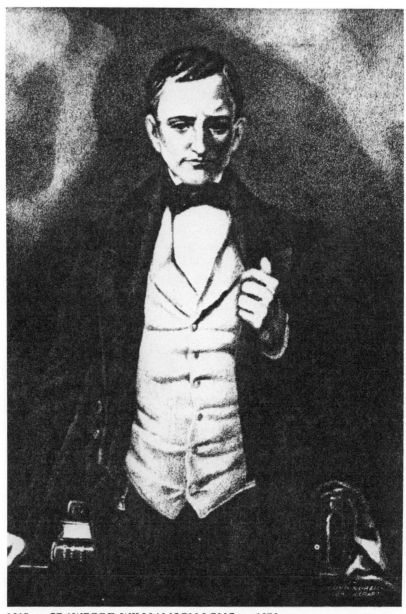

1815 — CRAWFORD WILLIAMSON LONG — 1878
The Discoverer of Anesthesia

NAME CHANGES TO CRAWFORD W. LONG MEMORIAL HOSPITAL

He giveth his beloved sleep.
Psalm 27.

Many accounts have been written of the achievement of Dr. Crawford Williamson Long, who discovered ether as a means of relieving patients of pain during surgery.

However, credit for this momentous change in the field of surgery long went unheralded.

The late Dr. Frank Kells Boland, Sr., a Crawford Long staff member, felt Long's achievement should be recognized. He devoted many years to verifying that Dr. Long was the discoverer and first user of ether as a general anesthetic. In 1926, Dr. Long's statue was placed in the Hall of Fame in Washington, D.C.

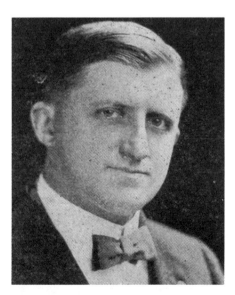

Dr. Frank K. Boland, author of THE FIRST ANESTHETIC, around 1926.

Dr. Fischer, who shared Dr. Boland's esteem for a fellow Georgia physician, also desired honor for Dr. Long. In an article he wrote for the May 2, 1937 Atlanta Constitution, Dr. Fischer explained why Dr. Long's name was chosen for the Davis-Fischer Sanatorium. "We decided to honor a long-departed member of our profession, Dr. Crawford Long, for his achievement in using sulphuric ether as an anesthetic for the first time on March 30, 1842. In selecting the name of Dr. Long as one that would be outstanding and would lend its influence to the future of the hospital, we felt the institution would continue to operate after the founders had grown tired of its operation or from the passing of years would be incapacitated to continue its active operation and that as time passed it would become more and more a public institution."

On March 30, 1931, as a part of the dedication of the newly-named hospital, a tablet and medallion of Dr. Long were unveiled in the presence of two of his daughters—Emma Long and Mrs. Eugenia Long Harper. The medallion bears Long's likeness in profile.

Two other tablets were unveiled that day. One in memory of Dr. Joseph Jacobs who was also instrumental in the effort to bring recognition to Dr. Long; the other tablet honored hospital founder Dr. E. C. Davis, who had recently died.

Sinclair Jacobs, Jr., grandson of Dr. Jacobs, unveiled the Jacobs' tablet. Sarah Fischer Davis and Theodore Lamar Davis, youngest children of Dr. Davis, uncovered the tablet of their father's likeness. Celebrated guests present at the ceremony were Governor L. H. Hardman, Chief Justice Richard B. Russell, Atlanta Mayor James L. Key, Dr. G. Y. Moore, President of the Georgia State Medical Association and Dr. F. C. Davison, President of the Fulton County Medical Society.

Mrs. A. R. Colcord, Regent of the Joseph Habersham Chapter and Mrs. Bun Wylie, State Regent of the Daughters of the American Revolution and Mrs. John A. Perdue, Honorary State President of the United Daughters of the Confederacy, were present to participate in the ceremony. Caroline Sutton, RN, Superintendent of the hospital, and Alice R. Thompson, President of the Davis-Fischer Sanatorium Alumni Association gave the pledge of loyalty to the institution.

The Rev. Richard Orme Flinn gave the invocation which was followed by an address by Rabbi David Marx. He praised Dr. Long as a "modest gentleman of the old school who exemplified the highest expression of kindness and loyalty of the ethics of the profession." He quoted Dr. Long's entry in his books on March 30, 1842: "For etherizing and incising of a tumor—$2.25."

Among medical dignitaries present from all over the country were Dr. E. G. Ballinger, who represented the Emory Unit, Base Hospital #43 of the AEF; Dr. Robert G. Stevens and Judge Alexander W. Stephens, grandson of Dr. Long's college roommate and classmate; and Dr. J. G. Ernest.

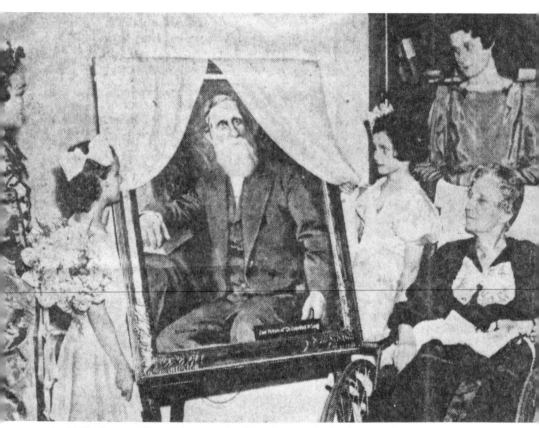

In 1935, the unveiling of the portrait of Dr. Long took place at Crawford Long as part of the observance of "Ether Day," commemorating the ninety-third anniversary of the discovery. Pictured are (left to right) Eulalia Vaughan, Margaret Dalton, Mary Brockman, Eleanor Miles, and Mrs. Eugenia Long Harper (in chair), daughter of the famous doctor. (Photo from the Atlanta Journal/ Constitution)

A BRIEF BIOGRAPHY OF DR. CRAWFORD LONG

Crawford Williamson Long, born on November 1, 1815 in Danielsville, Georgia, was the grandson of Revolutionary War soldiers of Irish ancestry. A quiet, studious boy who loved horses, fishing and sports, he entered Franklin College (now the University of Georgia) at age fourteen. While there, his roommate was Alexander H. Stephens, who later became governor of Georgia and vice-president of the Confederacy.

After graduation in 1835 with an A.M. degree, Long returned to Danielsville to teach school because his father considered him too young, at nineteen, to study medicine. He served as the principal of Danielsville Academy for one year and then he went to Jefferson, Georgia where he "read" medicine under the watchful eye of Dr. George R. Grant for a year. Following the prevailing custom, Long studied under the older physician, reading the doctor's books and picking up knowledge and skill by observing his teacher at work. He also studied at Transylvania Medical College in Kentucky. From there he enrolled at the Jefferson Medical College of the University of Pennsylvania. He was awarded a medical degree in 1839.

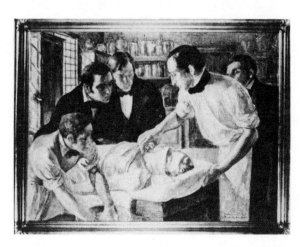

Artist's conception of the first anesthetic, March 30, 1842. Painted by Maurice Siegler.

As a medical student from a small country town, Long had observed with interest the "frolics" of fellow students. These were parties where nitrous oxide, known as "laughing gas" was inhaled for the momentary effect it produced. In his book, *Doctors on Horseback*, James Thomas Flexner wrote: "While a medical student in

Philadelphia, Long attended a chemical lecture during which a more up-to-date urban showman had induced drunkenness not with laughing gas but ether."

Long hurried home with his friends to their boarding house where they tried out the ether as an experiment. It worked! Even as he laughed at the ludicrous behavior of the men, he noticed that the students, first under the influence of nitrous oxide and then ether, did not complain of pain from cuts or bruises they received as they stumbled into the sharp corners of room furniture. Long asked them about this afterward. They insisted they felt nothing.

Long interned at hospitals in New York City. In 1841, he returned to Georgia and bought the practice of Dr. Grant, his former mentor. At that time, Georgia had a population of 517,000 persons, almost half of them slaves.

Dr. Long enjoyed the social life of his town, including laughing gas frolics. He pondered the lack of pain of those under the influence of ether, which gave a longer period of oblivion than laughing gas. It occurred to him that this could be more than a frivolous party pastime.

On March 30, 1842, when he was twenty-six years old, Dr. Long persuaded his friend James Venable to allow him to administer sulphuric ether to him so that a cyst on his neck could be excised. Four witnesses were present when the operation was successfully completed.

Dr. Long's purchase of the ether was recorded in Dr. Jacobs' pharmacy record book, which later was used to support his claim that he was the first to use ether as an anesthetic.

Four years after Dr. Long used ether, Dr. W. T. Morton, a Boston dentist, used ether for the extraction of a tooth at the suggestion of Dr. Charles Jackson, a chemist-scientist.

These two men colored ether and added aromatic oil flavoring to it and marketed it under the patented name "Lethon." Its sale was immediate to physicians and hospitals.

Dr. Long's use of ether on a cloth seems primitive. It was. Until Long's discovery, surgical operations were not only agonizing for the patient, they were taxing for the attending physician who had to work with lightning speed after his patient fainted from pain. Most surgery was confined to the outward body while assistants, strong enough to hold steady a tied-down patient, sweated as the doctor worked.

According to an account written by his daughter, Frances

Long Taylor, Dr. Long's first successful surgery was unintended.

When Dr. Long and his sister as children played a daredevil backyard game, she would snatch her fingers back before her brother could strike them with an ax. Suddenly, one day, her retraction was tardy. Down came the ax, slashing three of her fingers.

Although he was frightened, her brother stubbornly held the fingers in place until screams brought their mother to the scene. She dressed the wounds with sugar and bound up the hand. Mrs. Taylor said, in later days, her aunt's fingers were saved but remained forever scarred.

When Dr. Long married seventeen year old Mary Caroline Swain on August 11, 1842, he was late for the wedding ceremony because he was attending a patient. As soon as the ceremony was over, he left to resume treatment of that patient, leaving his bride to explain his absence to the guests. He returned the next day. And so it was for the rest of their wedded days. Dr. and Mrs. Long had twelve children. Two sons and three daughters reached adulthood.

The growing family moved to Atlanta in 1850 to live where present-day Broad and Luckie Streets meet. His office was in their home. Although Atlanta was young and smaller then, the Longs felt it was too crowded. They moved back to Jefferson, and later moved to Athens.

For a time, Dr. Long did nothing to let the world know of his discovery of the use of ether. However, when word came to him that others were claiming the discovery, he protested.

After a long and at times bitter controversy involving two dentists, Dr. Horace Wells and Dr. W. Morton, and a Dr. Jackson described by a contemporary as a "pertinacious and unscrupulous man who tried to purloin other people's inventions," Dr. Long was declared the legitimate discoverer.

Dr. Jackson admitted Dr. Long was the first man to use ether after he saw Dr. Jacobs' pharmacy record book and he had talked with witnesses to Venable's operation.

Morton, Wells, and Jackson each had claimed the discovery of ether. The conflict of who actually discovered it reached Congress in 1847. Then when the three fraudulent claimants had exhausted all their appeals, Georgia Senator W. C. Dawson arose to speak to Congress on April 15, 1854 naming Dr. Long as the genuine discoverer.

According to Dr. Boland in his researched and documented book: "This move is reported to have exploded a bombshell into the debate." The object of the dispute was two-fold; to determine who was the discoverer of anesthesia and mainly to decide who would receive the prize of $100,000, later raised to $200,000. The result of the war of words was that no prize was awarded.

As the rumbling of a coming crisis between the North and the South grew louder, Dr. Long opposed secession at first, even made a speech against it. But when Georgia left the Union, so did he. At 49, he enrolled as a private in Captain Taylor's Georgia Infantry Company.

When news came to his family that Union General Stoneman was approaching their home Athens, Frances Long remembered her father's command to guard a glass jar containing his papers that showed proof of his discovery of ether. She tied the jar to her waist with a rope and concealed it with her long skirt. The Confederates captured the advancing column of Union cavalry before it reached Athens.

When he was pressed into serving a Federal garrison stationed near Athens, he served to the best of his skill as a neutral agent of medicine. He was eventually appointed as the occupation encampments' chief surgeon. This service earned him a "pardon" from the United States Government, pardon for his participation in the War Between the States.

He was known as a man of honor. After the war's end, he paid the bill for medicine he had ordered from a northern firm, although the medicine was taken over for use by the Confederate Army. Not only did he pay for medicine he never received, he paid the interest on the bill.

Dr. Long lost much of his money during the war, but later again became prosperous. He treated patients far and wide, riding his horse Charley to isolated farmhouses where he often stayed for days at a time.

Dr. Jacobs, the pharmacist, later expressed his feeling for Dr. Long as his "example" and as one he loved as a father. He wrote: "Dr. Long was a quiet and unassuming man in deportment and address, gentle and gracious in manner with all whom he conversed, but with ever a retiring and modest means. He was particular in business dealings for just and honorable results and required order, cleanliness and system in all the appointments of the drugstore and office [owned by Dr. Long].

"His kindly disposition and quiet good humor attracted many friends to visit and exchange pleasantries when duty allowed a short respite."

Dr. Long occasionally wrote humorous sketches for the Athens newspaper "The Watchman" edited by John Christy. The sketches could be compared to a modern "roast" about friends whose names he changed to spare them open ridicule. They were, of course, recognized by his friends who laughed heartily at the jibes.

Dr. Long's daughter, writing of her father's last days, said, "My father's medical responsibilities seemed to grow heavier each day the last few months of his life. He was obliged to leave early in the morning, frequently not returning until late at night."

Of the last meal he shared with his family, she wrote: "He never seemed more interested or cheerful. Finally he grew serious and talked of life and its duties, then rising from the table he said with greatest gentleness and tenderness, 'No man ever had better children than I have.' "

To the end a healer, he safely delivered the wife of Congressman H. H. Carlton and then fell over on the bed. His last words were characteristic of his ever-present concern for a patient. "Care for the mother and child first." Then he collapsed. He was sixty-two years old.

Eight years after he died, in 1886, Mary Caroline Long wrote, in the style of her time, of her husband and his work: "We had prospered in this world's goods, had a lovely home and sweet, pleasant children, two sons and three daughters. My husband was the leading physician, fine-looking, a devoted husband and father, a kind judicious master [he had slaves prior to Civil War], beloved and respected by all classes. A large and lucrative practice enabled us to live handsomely, without entrenching on other sources of revenue. . . . Yes, we had an earthly paradise—that of perfect love and harmony.

"The laborious life of a village doctor, with an extensive practice in the adjoining country and villages and towns without railroads is hard to conceive now. To reach his patients, swollen streams had to be crossed at fords amid dangers, winter's cold and summer's heat disregarded, with loss of sleep and exhaustion the consequences . . . His ideals were noble and lofty, causing aspirations to make the most of himself for the good of mankind. For this he loved, labored, suffered and died."

Dr. Long practiced successfully for forty years. Today, his fame is worldwide. A bronze plaque honoring Dr. Long was placed in the Library of the Royal College of Surgeons in Edinburgh, Scotland by Mr. C. R. Nasmith, American Consul, on behalf of a group of American surgeons. In 1912, the University of Pennsylvania placed a medallion of Crawford Long to remind all who pass that he was an alumnus of that school.

On March 28, 1935, as part of a statewide Crawford Long Day exercise in Jefferson, a tablet was unveiled at the site of his office. Present were Dr. Hugh H. Young of Baltimore and Mrs. Eugenia Long Harper, Dr. Long's daughter. The marker was placed by the Works Progress Administration (WPA).

On September 15, 1957, the Crawford W. Long Memorial Museum in Jefferson was dedicated and opened to the public, in a building built before 1860 on the foundation of Dr. Long's original office.

The renaming of the Davis-Fischer Sanatorium in Atlanta in 1931 added lustre to Dr. Long's name and his name added prestige to Crawford W. Long Memorial Hospital.

Dr. Boland, who played a large part in keeping Dr. Long's name alive, died in November of 1953 after fifty years of medical practice and writing. From the "District Meter," 5th Georgia Nurses Association official publication of January 5, 1954, came these words:

"Dr. Boland, a warrior until the end, never gave up fighting for a cause he believed in and for many years he devoted his time to the verification and authorization of proper due credit to the name and fame of Georgia's Dr. Crawford Long as the discoverer and first user of ether as a general anesthesia. This he saw fulfilled with the erection of Dr. Long's statue in the Hall of Fame in Washington, D.C. and in the issuance of a postage stamp honoring him."

Dr. Boland's book, *The Story of Crawford Long—The First Anesthetic,* was published by the University of Georgia Press in 1950.

In the Crawford Long Nursing School records is a speech Dr. Boland made to the 1945 graduating class. Part of it says: "I wish to thank you for the splendid service you have given patients and the doctors and the hospital during the time you spent here. You notice I mention patients first because they should always receive first attention.

"The hospital here bears the name of Georgia's most distinguished physician wisely and appropriately given it by Dr. Fischer fifteen years ago. This name is also your charge, and I know you will guard and protect it zealously and sacredly."

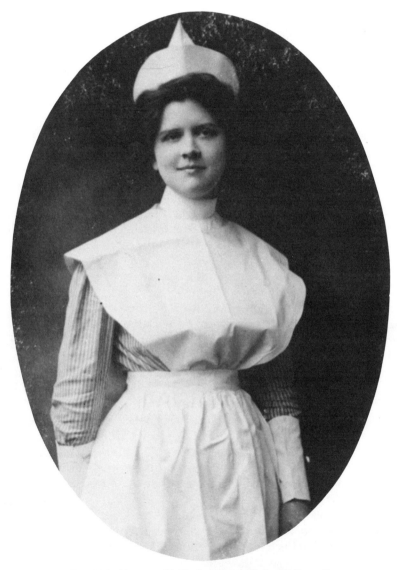

*In 1911, 22 year old Gladys Marshall Smith Barnett
was one of three members of the first graduating
class of the School of Nursing.*

CHAPTER   THREE

NURSING
EDUCATION

In 1842, when Dr. Crawford Long administered ether as an anesthetic for the first time, trained nurses did not exist.

With the introduction of female nurses on the battlefields of the Civil War, a precedent was set. The women, their abilities proven, came home determined to get a foothold in civic institutions to give humane care to the sick. It wasn't easy for them. Change came slowly.

In Georgia, modern nurse training started about the turn of the century, and the rules for those pioneer nurses were stiff. Everyday, the nurse swept and mopped the floor of her ward, dusted and took care of linens. To keep an even temperature in the ward for her many patients, she was to bring in coal during cold weather. She also was required to fill all lamps with kerosene, clean the chimneys and trim wicks. Windows were to be washed once a week. When she made out reports, she was to make quill pens carefully but could whittle nibs to her own taste. Steel pens were allowed.

She reported to duty at 7 a.m. and worked until 8 p.m., except on Sunday, when she was free from noon until 2 p.m. Graduate nurses in good standing were allowed an evening off each week if they attended church. If she earned $80 a month, she was expected to set aside $15 for her old age. Any nurse who used tobacco or alcohol, had her hair dressed at a beauty parlor, or went to dance halls would be in trouble.

A nurse who was attentive and served her patients and physicians faithfully and faultlessly for five years was to receive a raise of five cents per day—providing the hospital had no outstanding debts.

Gradually, things changed. Dr. Frank Boland, in an address to the Crawford Long 1943 graduating class, said: "Remember that skill in bedside care is still the heart of the nursing profession. We are fond of referring to Florence Nightingale as the mother of nursing, as indeed she was, but she knew nothing of aseptic surgery or of the many other things you are required to know."

Outstanding achievements of the graduates of Crawford Long Nursing School have been a source of pride over its entire history. When the Davis-Fischer Sanatorium began treating patients, it also began training nurses, with a class of seven young women eager to work and learn. There were no entrance requirements other than ambition. Three of these young women graduated in 1911.

Back then, an aspiring nurse was interviewed by the training superintendent, Lou Miller, who had come to Atlanta from Chicago's Mercy Hospital. The applicant was then sent to Dr. Davis for final approval. When that was given, she was placed in a class. Since training consisted of learning by doing and practically no book work, the student donned a uniform, covered it with a large wrap-around apron and began rounds with the superintendent. She shared with the doctor complete responsibility for patient care.

When Anna Brundage became Superintendent of Nurses in the Sanatorium's second year, she started student lectures by practicing doctors—when they were available. If the lecturer was detained by a case, the class was dismissed. This was the beginning of academic education, along with bedside training.

Miss Brundage was succeeded by Lillian Joselyn, also from Chicago's Mercy Hospital. She upgraded the training program by requiring two years of high school for trainees. She also eased some of the strict rules.

Hours of duty were shortened. Student nurses not on duty were allowed to stay out until eleven o'clock once a week but were required to be in their quarters by 9 p.m. the other nights. Overnight leaves were unknown except for annual vacations.

Upon graduation, the girls automatically became RNs.

In 1915, Agnes McGinley redesigned the school's nurse's cap. She also improved living conditions in the residence on the corner of West Peachtree and Linden, where fireplaces provided heat and hot baths were on a "first come, first served" basis.

In World War I, nurses from Davis-Fischer joined the Emory Unit which served in France. Dr. Davis organized the group of physicians, enlisted men and one hundred nurses who reported to the Davis-Fischer Sanatorium in March 1918 for transport to Camp Gordon, and eventually overseas.

That year, Caroline Sutton, a Davis-Fischer graduate, became the hospital's Superintendent of Nurses. Clare Swanson served as her assistant. Nurses were now being assigned to specialty services and were rotated as ordered.

In 1921, the Georgia legislature passed a law that required all graduate nurses to pass a State Board Examination before they could affix RN (Registered Nurse) after their names. Nurses who'd already graduated could no longer use RN.

Graduates were indignant but the law stayed. However, a concession was made. A five-dollar fee was imposed and a five-day moratorium was declared, thus giving graduated nurses five days to register without examination. Undergraduates had to abide by the new law.

A handwritten caption identifies these women as the School of Nursing Class of 1926. They are Sarah Murray, Kathryn Sylvester, Ruth Harrison, Natalie Johnson, Floye Christian, Thelma Tallent, Edna Collins, Jewell Poore, Louise Curtis, Ethel Moffet, Edna Carmicheal, Mary Lee, Grace Scroggins, Lura Hurst, Mozelle Christian, Louise McArthur.

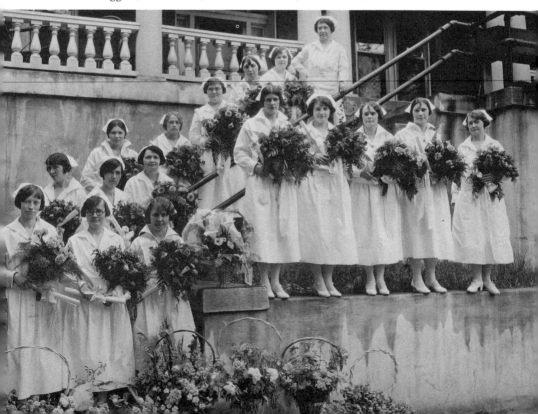

In the "roaring twenties," Dr. Fischer tolerated raised hems of the students' blue and white striped uniforms but balked at bobbed hair. The first nurse who appeared with clipped locks was fired! However, the tearful girl appealed to Dr. Davis. The father of five daughters, Dr.Davis was aware of current styles. He conferred with Dr. Fischer, and the nurse was reinstated.

Miss Sutton continued as Superintendent of Nurses until 1927, when Alice Thompson succeeded her.

The 1929 stock market crash and the Great Depression had its impact on the Davis-Fischer Sanatorium and all hospitals.

Nurses were thrown out of work when people couldn't pay for medical treatment. More and more hospital beds remained empty. With regret, Dr. Fischer closed the Nurse's Training School on March 28, 1932 to cut down on the number of nurses graduating into the scarce employment situation generated by hard times.

In a letter to another doctor, Dr. Fischer wrote that hospital fees had been lowered "to help the men of modest means through the present economic condition." He set a fixed rate of $25 for five days of hospitalization for the wives of men in need during the birth of a child.

Times got better, and classes resumed in 1936. In 1939, the first class of the reopened School of Nursing graduated twelve nurses. The program continued to expand. Ruth Babin became Superintendent of Nurses in 1941 and it was during her tenure that the new nurses' home on West Peachtree Street was built.

Charge for admission to the School of Nursing increased to $50. A systematic rotation for specialty work was established and pediatric nursing was taught at Egleston Hospital for Children. College courses at the Georgia School of Business Administration were added to the curriculum.

Eventually, admission requirements included a high school diploma earned by passing grades in fifteen units of English, mathematics, social studies, and science or foreign language. Students were required to present evidence of personal and physical fitness.

The five aims of the three-year school were to educate nurses to give skilled and intelligent care, to teach recognition of the patient as an individual, to teach others the principles and practice of health and disease prevention, to guide the students to well-adjusted personalities, to make them capable of adjusting to changing situations, and to develop their own capacities as individuals.

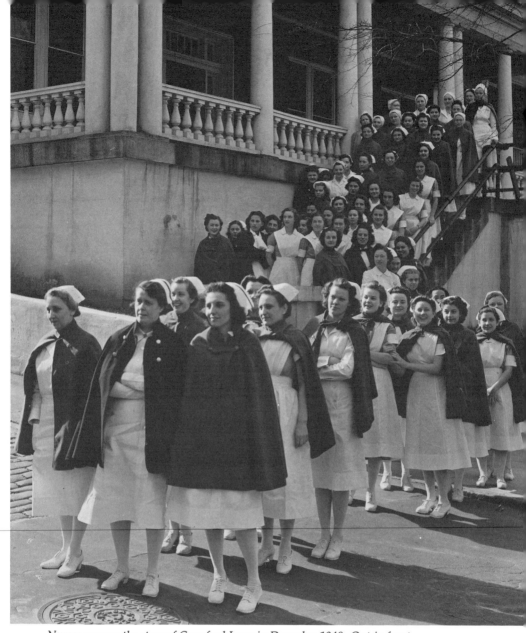

Nurses pose on the steps of Crawford Long in December 1940. Out in front are (left to right) Macie S. Stephens, Director of Nursing, Edna Morgan, Director of Nursing Education, and Miss Miriani, an instructor.

By 1947, when May Sanders was Director of Nursing, class size had expanded to meet the growing need for nurses. In 1949, Ruth Babin was again Director of Nursing, with Georgia B. Hearn Martin as her assistant. Jeanne Lambie followed Miss Babin, who was succeeded by Macie Stephens, a Crawford Long graduate.

Dr. Shelley Davis said of her, "There is hardly a department that has not felt the helpful and guiding touch of Mrs. Stephens. Doctors and patients alike cherish her friendship, and student nurses rely on her unselfish judgment, love and her dedication to service."

In May 1961, Evangeline Lane, Director of Nursing Education at Crawford Long, announced the rule against married students was being relaxed. Prior to this time, student nurses were forbidden to marry until the last six months of the three-year training. The rule caused a large dropout in the number of student nurses each year. The rule change came at a time when there was an acute nurse shortage due to the building of many new hospitals. Married students were allowed to live off campus, another first.

In July of 1960, a fine student confessed she had secretly married. The faculty, after careful consideration, decided to let her stay in school. Thus, Crawford Long Hospital became the first nursing school in the area to accept married students. Mrs. Lane said then, "Dr. Glenn approved of marriage and maternity. The married girl stayed on."

Although this change of policy wasn't publicized, two marriages followed in the spring. Married students from other hospitals transferred to Crawford Long, to be followed by still others. To meet the inevitable, a maternity uniform was designed. The joyful young women termed it "adorable."

Through the 1950s, seventy percent of America's nurses came out of three-year hospital diploma courses like Crawford Long's. The balance came from college programs.

By this time, wards were called units. It was no longer considered necessary for a student nurse to have her hair clipped or pinned higher than her uniform collar. Wash and wear uniforms replaced stiffly starched dresses and aprons. Motherhood was not a hindrance to training.

Pat Adams came to nursing school a little later in life than most of the students. When her daughter Lori was born at Crawford Long, Mrs. Adams became inspired to become a nurse. When Lori was eighteen months old, her mother enrolled, graduating in 1970. Like so many Crawford Long graduates, she stayed at her "own hospital" where she herself had been born and was trained.

When Pat Adams was chosen as the September 1972 Employee of the Month, she said, "I love nursing and I love Floor 4-C. I will stay here forever if they will let me."

The Crawford Long School of Nursing gained recognition

for an historical display entered in the 1979 Powers Crossroads Country Fair and Arts Festival. Their exhibition took first prize in the education category.

The authentic display showed historical medical equipment and uniforms and highlighted information about Crawford Long Hospital and its Nursing School. Ann Stroud, Director of Nursing Education, was the coordinator for the display viewed by thousands. Student nurses, under the direction of Glendora Robinson, the nursing history teacher, dressed fifty dolls in copies of uniforms that nurses have worn over the years.

During "Stay and See Georgia Week" held at Lenox Square in July 1979, the Crawford Long students' display again won first prize in the education category. Over half a million people saw the display of medical equipment and uniforms and received information about the school.

Katherine Pope, present Assistant Administrator for Nursing Service, has been both an eyewitness and a participant in the expansion of Crawford Long Hospital, dating back to 1958 when she came to work at Crawford Long at the invitation of Macie Stephens. Her assignment was to teach Communicable Disease Nursing and Orthopedics in the School of Nursing, utilizing her teaching experience at Grady Hospital.

At first she was a part-time worker and a student at Georgia State University. Later, Mrs. Stephens and Dr. Glenn asked Miss Pope to become Acting Director of Nurses. "I did agree to help them," she said as she recalled work with Dr. Glenn as a student nurse at Grady when he served as Associate Professor of Surgery. "I had operated with Dr. Glenn and worked with him as Administrative Assistant at Grady, working with him and other surgeons for planning the areas of the new hospital. I did make the stipulation that I continue my nursing education which both he and Mrs. Stephens supported." Miss Pope served as Acting Director of Nurses until January of 1970. During her time of service, Miss Pope and Mrs. Evangeline Lane, Director of Nursing Education, met weekly with Dr. Glenn to discuss the Nursing Program and plan for student educational advancement.

In 1960, anesthesiologists took on the task of respiratory therapy, which nurses had handled in the past. Until that time, the hospital employed clinical dietitians, but very few other technical workers.

Miss Pope said, "The emergence of so many technicians and

the addition of physical therapists, social services, utilization review nurses, urodynamic technicians, vascular technicians and physician's assistants changed the picture. All these new kinds of workers, directly and indirectly involved in patient care, caused complication in the coordination of patient care.

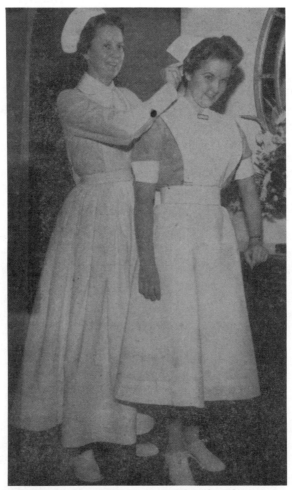

Katherine Pope in 1961 as she and Martha Johnson demonstrate the changes in nurses' uniforms over the fifty years between 1911 (Miss Pope's uniform) and 1961 (Miss Johnson's uniform). (Photo from Atlanta Journal/Constitution)

"We have tried to hold on [what] that we truly see as nursing. . . . We think our Career Advancement Program assisted us in this."

Miss Pope recalls Dr. Glenn's approval of reduced duty hours for nurses from forty-four to forty hours a week as an incentive to retain professional nurses. "Dr. Glenn also authorized us to employ part-time nurses as well as to create a pool of these staff members. Twenty years later, this became the vogue in the nursing profession. But it became a commercial pool in which institutions had to pay the agencies for similar resources that we created within our Nursing Department in the early 1960s.

"Fortunately, Crawford Long never had to utilize commercial resource pools which were far more costly to the institution and to the patients. Those innovations had, as the key factor, Dr. Glenn's understanding of the concept that ultimately helped us keep nurses in the practice of nursing."

She remembers the period from 1960-1970 as one that filled the hospital beds and sometimes overflowed to patient beds in the corridors, but needs were met.

When other hospitals declined to receive patients from the Florence Crittenton organization caring for unwed mothers, Crawford Long administrators, after an hour's discussion, agreed to accept the mothers-to-be for delivery of their babies.

Mrs. Pope recalls the first Home Health Care Nurse at the hospital was assigned to Crawford Long in the mid-60s in a part-payment agreement with the Atlanta Community Council. "This program became a model for the community."

When Katherine Pope left Crawford Long in January 1970 to pursue a Masters degree, she was honored with a farewell reception. Dr. Glenn presented her with a silver tray and words of thanks for her eleven years of service engraved on its back. He recalled their work together at the Steiner Clinic at Grady Hospital and his request that she come to work at Crawford Long.

At that time, Miss Pope told the story of a man whose wife died at Crawford Long, leaving him four small children and a large hospital bill.

"He didn't have any insurance," she said. "So the hospital allowed him to pay by the month, interest-free at a rate he could afford.

"Just before Christmas one year, when all but $1,000 had been paid, the hospital notified the man that the benefactor fund of the hospital would pay the remaining $1,000. That is the sort of thing that has touched me most about being at Crawford Long," she said. "It's not the physical plant—it's the people that are important.

"I was away five years but never truly 'away' in that Mr. Barker and I served on many committees and I continued to work with Nursing staff members. Crawford Long was like home to me. Often I was in contact with the nursing family. I also stayed in touch with Dr. Glenn. I was involved with the State Planning Commission which Governor Carter established and when that project terminated, I was exploring positions." When Dr. Glenn and Mr. Barker learned this, they invited her to return to Crawford Long.

She "came home" in September of 1975, at the time many nurses were moving out of the City of Atlanta into adjoining counties. This sorely affected downtown institutions' personnel needs. Downtown hospitals, acutely short-staffed, turned to recruiting foreign nurses.

Miss Pope brought with her a belief that the inner city would rebuild and Crawford Long Hospital, so long a part of Atlanta, would survive and continue to serve downtown and the surrounding community.

"The downtown community is revitalizing, has survived," said Miss Pope in 1986. "From a nursing perspective, the greatest thing on my return to Crawford Long was that so many of my colleagues had stayed in downtown Atlanta. That group joined to focus on what we needed to do to help the nursing program to continue."

Crawford Long nurses reviewed the report of the National Information Study. A Task Force was formed; it recommended a Career Advancement Program for the nurses who practice at Crawford Long.

"We have created a program in which the staff members practice nursing as they are educated, as they work they continue to learn and grow. We believe that what we have been able to put together has served not only our patient community but also our profession around the country." This program became a model for the nation. Crawford Long's program was described in the October 1981 issue of American Journal of Nursing.

In 1982 the program concepts were presented to the ANA Biannual meeting. Subsequently, the Cabinet of Nursing Service published a statement on the Career Advancement Program. Both the ANA staff and Cabinet used the model for illustration of information regarding career advancements.

Concerning the Career Advancement Program, Miss Pope said, "I think the roles of Medical Director and Administrator were significant in the patient programs and in the nursing efforts. Always upon presentation of the program the question arose as to how we would sell it to Administration. I wish the record to reflect that it never was a problem with our Medical Director and Administrator. They had an interest and gave us support and input that aided us in having the best of programs."

Miss Pope traveled to China twice to share her knowledge. As a member of the People to People Delegation invited by the China Association of Science and Technology and the China Nurses Association, she traveled throughout China for three weeks in the spring of 1982. During this time she shared the Career Advancement Program and her experience in the restructuring of the Nursing Service Program.

In the spring of 1985, she returned to China to present a paper on Crawford Long's Neonatal Program as a part of the United States Scientific China Presentation for Medical Nursing Exchange. At this time, she was asked how an intensive care program for infants might be established.

She drew on her experience with the updated Crawford Long Nursery and her work with the nursing staff and nurse practitioners. "We have pretty much become a model for the community in use of nurse practitioners with established protocols in which these qualified nurses are in-house to provide constant neonate support. With them we are able to care for more neonates."

Miss Pope, proud of the progress of nursing at Crawford Long and her part in it, said, "I think we would be remiss if we did not recognize that for many years Crawford Long was the obstetrical training center of this region. Our nursing education program and our experience in the nursing service reveals this hospital is a community, a family community. If you are a member of the Crawford Long Hospital Employee group, you are a member of the family. This hospital, as a family, has served this city and its citizens."

Over time, as new academic programs emerged in the community, the faculty of the Crawford Long School proposed and received Board of Nursing accreditation for an educational curriculum change, setting the trend for hospital schools of nursing. The changes implemented supported the continuation of hospital schools of nursing for a period of time.

But nursing education, like other professions has expanded in colleges and universities, while the number of hospital schools of nursing has decreased dramatically. Because of this trend, it was decided the CWL School of Nursing would close after the June 1988 graduation of the class that entered in September 1985. The Crawford Long Nursing School has educated approximately two thousand nurses.

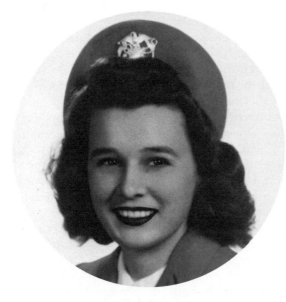

Helon Burton Seigler,
a Cadet Nurse
during World War II,
is still on duty
at Crawford Long.

CADET NURSE PROGRAM

Mrs. Helon Burton Seigler, RN, is a graduate of the Crawford Long School of Nursing and was a Cadet Nurse in the Corps formed during World War II.

The Cadet Corp began in 1940. The possibility of United States entering the war in Europe began a push to recruit more registered nurses.

In July of 1940, the Nursing Council for National Defense included six nursing organizations (ANA, NLNE, NOPHN, ACSN, NACGN and AAIW), the Federal Nursing Service and representatives from the American Hospital Association. Later, the name became the National Nursing Council for War Services.

When many RNs, including several from Crawford Long, enlisted in the Armed Services, the National Nursing Council rallied to plan recruiting students for nursing schools to replace the departing women.

Consequently, a plan was proposed to the United States government for funds to finance such a program. There were delays, but in June 1941, a law was passed providing $1,200,000 to assist in training nurses that fiscal year. In July of 1942, the federal appropriation was increased to $3.5 million. In 1943, a bill sponsored by Congresswoman Frances Payne Bolton asked for $60 million. The Bolton Act created the United States Cadet Nurse Corps.

Miss Helon Burton left her job as a high school French teacher to train at Crawford Long Hospital as a cadet. This is her account of her participation in that program now a part of WWII history.

"During the World War II days, the Crawford W. Long School of Nursing became a member of the Cadet Nurse Corps.

"The Corps was a federally funded nurse training program designed to relieve the 'nurse shortage'—to provide more nurses for the 'Armed Forces' and to staff the 'at home hospitals.' "

"Established in 1943, it provided for a thirty-month basic program, free tuition and fees, free uniforms, monthly stipends ($60 per month by the senior year, I think!) for the students in approved Schools of Nursing." Approved schools were required to meet standards developed by the National League of Nursing Education (NLNE).

Students who entered the program pledged to serve where needed in military or civilian agencies for the duration of the war and six months thereafter. By the end of the war, cadet nurses numbered 179,000.

Forty years later, seven former cadet nurses were employed at Crawford Long Hospital—six of them are graduates of Crawford Long School of Nursing. Helon Burton Seigler, Virginia Benefield, Marian Taylor, Margaret Fowler, Juanita Linkous, Katherine Pope, and Anna Belle Ivey are former "cadets."

"Crawford Long was admitting classes every three months when I entered in 1944. Ninety-four seniors graduated in 1947.

"The educational program we followed was structured but not 'military' in any way except one attempt at 'teaching us military bearing.'

"Off duty, we proudly wore cadet nurse uniforms—very attractive suits. A cotton summer uniform of gray and white pinstripe with red epaulets. A winter uniform of gray wool with red epaulets and a 'tam' (hat!).

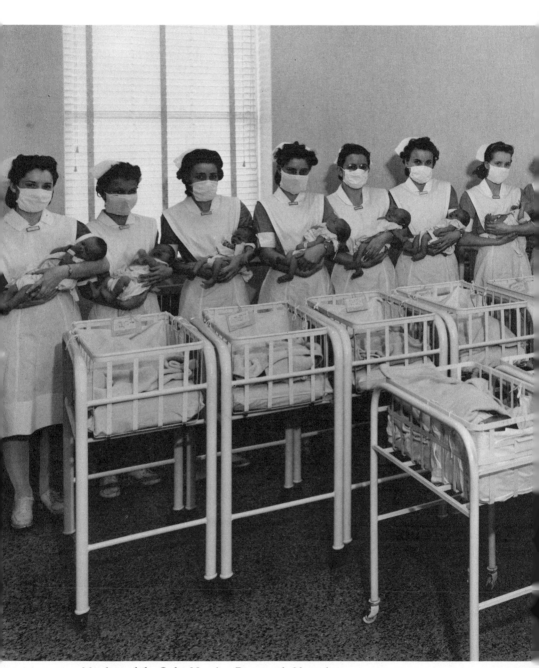

Members of the Cadet Nursing Program hold newborns.

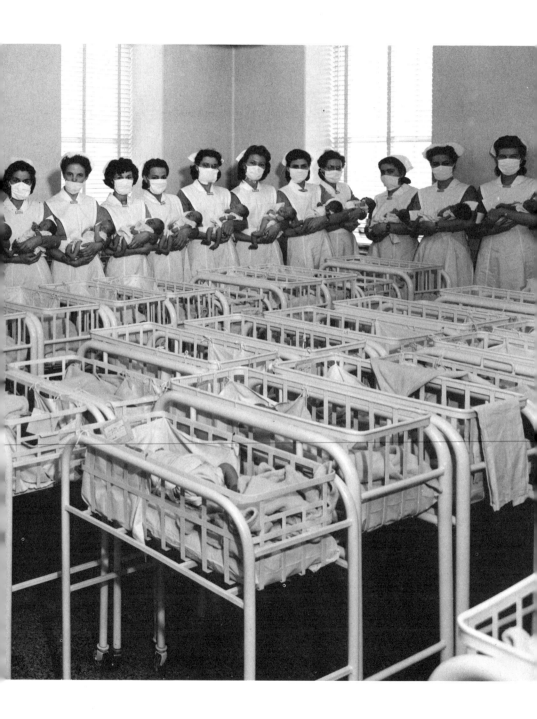

"One day during our freshman year, we donned our uniforms per order, 'marched' to the Marist Drill Field to 'drill.' As I recall, a Marine sergeant had the dubious honor of 'shaping' up the student nurses.

"At the end of the first afternoon, he gave the order 'right face'—half of us promptly turned right and the other half turned left! That was the end of our military experience.

"We never knew what happened to the Marine sergeant . . .

"We attended classes and staffed the hospital during the war years. Most of the registered nurses had joined the war effort. The only RNs left were supervisors (five to cover all three shifts) and one registered nurse per operating room to teach students how to scrub.

"We loved working in the Operating Room. No one complained about scrubbing from 7 a.m. until midnight, if needed. As the supply of interns and residents was also scanty, we frequently served as assistants to the surgeons.

"Seniors were head nurses on the floors (units) and student nurses served as their staff. There were no LPNs, nursing assistants, unit clerks, respiratory therapists, physical therapists, therapeutic dietitians. Student nurses, plus an orderly, provided all the patient care.

"Crack an oxygen tank. Blow an electric fan (yes, we *did* have electricity) over a pan of ice to cool craniotomy patients with 105 degree temperatures. Make cotton balls. Boil syringes and needles. File 'burrs' from hypodermic needles. Wash and powder rubber gloves. Set up sterile trays in Central Service. Prepare special diets.

"Whatever the patient needed, we provided. Then, as now, nurses were caring, committed, and competent. And our patients loved us. 'The best nurses in Atlanta are at Crawford Long Hospital' was common knowledge. To us, our duty was to care for our patients in every way and we never questioned it.

"It was, therefore, a definite shock to the four of us who went to New York City to complete the last six months of our education to find that *our* quality of nursing was not universal.

"One of the fringe benefits of the cadet program was that the senior nurse could complete the last six months of her training at any hospital she chose. So, four of us headed for New York City. Two others selected Johns Hopkins. We were assigned to hospitals on Welfare Island in the middle of the East River.

"Within one month of our arrival, we CWL students were assigned as head nurses of wards and permitted to work in the research units of Goldwater Geriatric Hospital [the first geriatric hospital]. We were the only affiliates selected for these prestigious assignments . . .

"All of us returned to Crawford Long. Mary Snow who had studied preemie care at Johns Hopkins was instrumental in developing the first premature nursery in this area [in 1947]. Essie Strickland Nugent later became an Administrator in the American Red Cross.

"And I (who joyfully abandoned the teaching profession forever when I joined the Cadet Nurse Corps) dutifully agreed to teach medical-surgical nursing to sixty students.

"Nursing instructors remained in the classrooms, never worked with the students on the floors. However, I was permitted, when not in the classroom, to work with the students on the floors on any shift—on my own time, of course. After all, I was earning $162 per month."

That's how Helon Seigler began providing clinical supervision in person. Today, she is Quality Assurance Nursing Service Coordinator at Crawford Long.

Miss Alice Thompson, Director of Nursing, smiles at a newborn.

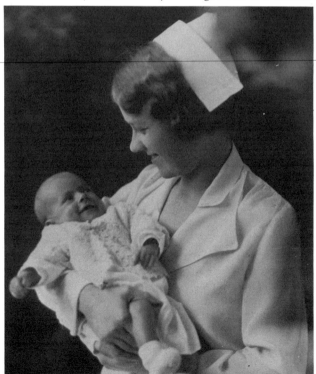

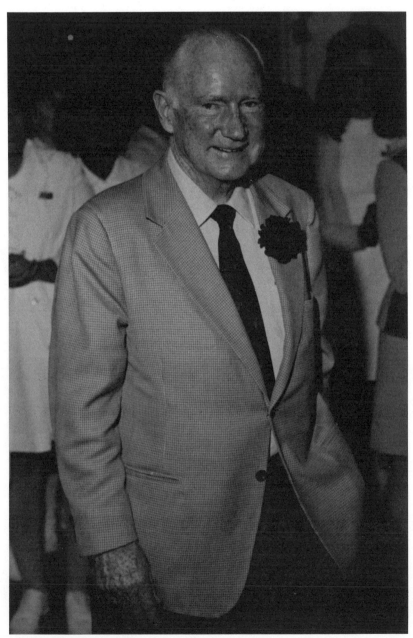

Dr. Wadley Raoul Glenn

DR. WADLEY RAOUL GLENN

When Dr. Fischer died in 1953, the members of the Emory Board of Trustees agreed as one that Dr. Wadley R. Glenn, who had served as the Crawford Long Medical Director since 1946, was the man to succeed Dr. Fischer.

Dr. Glenn's capacity to cope and succeed was acclaimed in the diamond anniversary brochure (published in 1983), "75 Years of Caring in Atlanta."

The first page told of Dr. Glenn's ability to relate to people. It said, "The one man whose contribution and influence has been exceptionally significant in bringing Crawford Long to its present level of excellence is Dr. Wadley R. Glenn, and it is to him that we dedicate this diamond anniversary publication.

"For more than forty years Dr. Glenn has given Crawford Long his wisdom as an administrator, his skill as a physician and his example as a leader.

"Some 2,400 years ago Hippocrates wrote, 'For where there is love of man there is love of art.' And so it is with Dr. Glenn. His love for humankind produces a desire to give the best of himself as well as to insure that the hospital meets the highest standards in every way. In accomplishing his objectives Dr. Glenn projects the quiet strength and singular determination typical of those who are sure of their direction and certain of its worthiness.

"He is an astute business manager, an outstanding planner but most endearing and impressive to all who know him is his gentle and compassionate spirit."

Wadley Raoul Glenn was born in Atlanta on February 6, 1905, three years before the Davis-Fischer Sanatorium began treating patients. In 1908, Wadley Glenn's father, Thomas K. Glenn, was made president of the Atlantic Steel Company.

Thomas K. Glenn, noted financier and philanthropist, contributed much to Atlanta. The family name appears on the Glenn Memorial United Methodist Church at Emory University in honor of Dr. Glenn's grandfather, the Rev. Wilbur F. Glenn, a Methodist minister who served as a chaplain in the Confederate Army. The Agnes Raoul Glenn Memorial Building at Crawford Long Hospital bears the name of Dr. Glenn's mother, who died when he was nine years old. The Thomas K. Glenn Building at Grady Memorial Hospital was named in honor of Dr. Glenn's father.

The young Wadley Glenn enrolled at Georgia Institute of Technology in the 1924 freshman class. James A. Hayes, an Atlanta real estate broker who was a classmate, said, "Wadley was popular and prominent on campus. In addition to his winsome manner, Wadley enjoyed many advantages. He was a native of Atlanta, the scion of a wealthy and prominent family, a good fraternity man and member of various social societies. In his freshman and sophomore years he was on the swimming team, winning laurels with the breast stroke."

Mr. Hayes said with a grin, "The only unlaudatory thing said about him was in the *Blue Print* [Georgia Tech Annual] in our freshman year. He was therein listed as 'W. R. Gleen.' He overcame that!"

The 1928 *Blue Print* carried the information that Wadley Glenn was a member of the Kappa Sigma Fraternity, Koseme, Bull Dogs, Skull and Key, and the Cotillion Club. He was also a member of the swimming team, football manager and a member of the American Society of Mechanical Engineers and the Student Council. He attained the rank of lieutenant of the ROTC.

After graduating from Georgia Tech, he worked for a year as an engineer for the Georgia Power Company at Tugalo Dam. He went back to school, enrolling in the Emory University School of Medicine. Graduating with honors, he served his internship and residency in surgery at Grady Hospital before joining the Emory University faculty to teach surgery.

While he was a senior medical student at Emory, he met Frances Lewis of Cairo, Georgia. She was a nurse at Grady Hospital and became his wife. Mrs. Glenn said of their wartime courtship and marriage, "It was not dull. At the outbreak of World War II, Dr. Glenn joined the Navy and was stationed at Camp Gordon in Chamblee. After Pearl Harbor, he was transferred to Pensacola Naval Air Station where he trained as a flight surgeon.

"We had dated regularly since 1935 so when he could not get leave to come to Atlanta, I flew to Pensacola and we were married at the Methodist parsonage. After three months, we were transferred back to Georgia to the Naval Station at Chamblee. After a year there, we were transferred to Cherry Point, North Carolina and stayed there over a year."

Then Dr. Glenn's Unit, 33rd Air Wing, was ordered to the Pacific. In the meantime, Mrs. Glenn drove to California to join her husband, only to learn that his unit had moved to Eagle Mountain Lake, Texas. So she drove to Texas, where the young couple lived for four months until he was ordered overseas.

Mrs. Glenn drove back to Atlanta. Then, a phone call from Lt. Glenn, asking her to join him in San Diego for the time before he left for the combat zone, sent her crow-hopping by airplane to California. "After being bumped quite a few times," she said, "I arrived in San Diego. In a few weeks, he went to the South Pacific and was there for over a year."

Somehow, despite censored mail, Mrs. Glenn had the impression her husband thought he wouldn't survive combat. "I had no idea where he was," she said. "And I missed him and worried about his return in that time when many of our friends did not make it."

Dr. Glenn was aboard the battleship *Missouri* where the peace treaty with Japan was signed in September 1945. He was discharged as a U.S. Navy Commander. Mrs. Glenn said, "He came back to Atlanta to resume his life's work, giving his all to the betterment of the people, never being too busy to listen to and help others less fortunate. It seems ironic that the disease he had worked so hard to help find a cure for was the final cause of his death."

Mrs. Glenn said she "always thought that Wadley went into medicine because of his mother's death from a tumor in 1914. In Wadley's last years, he would often go to the Grady Hospital Clinic. He had a great interest in this subject. I can't say for sure, but I've often thought this was why he went into medicine."

After Dr. Glenn returned from the war, the couple moved into the family home, Glenridge Hall, which was built in 1929 by Dr. Glenn's father on land purchased in 1912. "We lived there for five years; meanwhile our daughter, Frances, and our son, Raoul, were born," she said. After the Glenns built themselves a smaller house on the property, their son Kearney was born.

Mrs. Glenn said, "I understood when we were married that

as a physician, he would be gone much of the time; we couldn't always do as we wanted. I busied myself with the children and my needlepoint. I was perfectly willing to remain in the background as his work at the hospital took more and more of his time and energy."

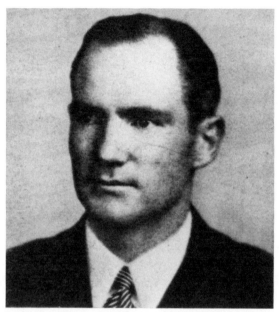

Dr. Glenn's photo from 1947 edition of The Phenap.

Horseback riding was a favorite family pastime at that time when family members could ride all the way to the Chattahoochee River and all around Dunwoody and never see a car.

Speaking again of her husband's work, Mrs. Glenn said, "I think Dr. Glenn's work at Crawford Long was worthwhile. It is what he set out to do and he did it. The hospital was his whole life. I felt he knew what he was doing, that it was what he wanted to do. I was willing for this. He did things I didn't know about, as he was quiet, but other people told me about them. I knew he went to work at Grady every Saturday morning but he didn't discuss such things much."

Under Dr. Glenn's leadership, many new services became a part of Crawford Long's outreach: the area's first blood bank, the first premature baby nursery, the establishment of a nuclear medi-

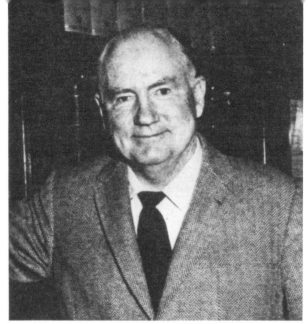

Dr. Glenn smiles from the pages of The Phenap, *1966.*

cine unit in the early 1960s, and the development of the Carlyle Fraser Heart Center for the diagnosis and treatment of coronary disease.

During Dr. Glenn's forty years at Crawford Long, much was written by him and about him. In the 1985 special edition of the Crawford Long newsletter "Larynx," dedicated to Dr. Glenn, it was said, "He could be seen almost any hour of the day, any day of the week. He calls his employees by name whether they have been there thirty-six years or two."

Dr. Glenn's keen interest in Crawford Long's workers never flagged. Through the years his column, "From the Director," praised staff members, encouraged them to strive for excellence and personal satisfaction. No phase of Crawford Long's operation was overlooked in his endeavor to provide quality care to its patients. Over and over he pointed out that quality of service was the ultimate goal of the Crawford Long family of workers.

He kept personnel feeling positive over new building construction by pointing out that frustrating happenings were a temporary inconvenience that would soon be forgotten when the new building became "home."

He could be firm when an occasion required firmness. Bill Moore, Director of Engineering Service at Crawford Long, became acquainted with Dr. Glenn in 1947. With a smile he said, "After I came to work here in 1974, Dr. Glenn would say to me, 'Now I want you to do a little job. There is no big hurry.' I understood he wanted it to be done as soon as possible, and it was. He was kind but firm. I never knew of a time he was wrong. I don't know of anyone who didn't have utmost regard for him."

Dr. Glenn's engineering training at Georgia Tech and his work on the Tugalo Dam project provided him with technical and nuts-and-bolts knowledge of the functioning of sections of the hospital that aren't seen by the public. Boiler, laundry and machine rooms of the hospital complex, with its tunnels and offices, corridors and elevators, patient beds and waiting rooms, cafeteria and communication network—even the beauty shop—were familiar walkways to Dr. Glenn. The people who worked there were familiar with his twinkling eyes, his friendly greetings and the scope of his knowledge about their tasks.

Dr. Glenn had a talent for bringing out the best in everyone who worked at the hospital, and he challenged them to recruit workers like themselves, people he called "the cream of the crop." "Tell them about the hospital," he wrote. "About the congenial atmosphere that abounds here."

Ever thoughtful, Dr. Glenn thanked employees for overcoming hardships caused by a bus strike in July of 1973, complimenting those who went out of their way to pick up stranded workers or went after others who needed transportation. He wrote in the Larynx, "Here is another example of why Crawford Long is known as a hospital that cares about its patients and its employees. Our hospital family united in amost admirable way to meet the emergency." As an example, he told of Gladys Avery who arranged for a taxi to bring her to work each morning. Ordinarily, Mrs. Avery, a twenty-two year housekeeping employee, boarded a bus at 5:20 a.m. so she could start her work by 6 a.m.

Jack Abbott, Assistant Director of Data Processing, recalls a remark by Dr. Jim Olley, Director of Pathology, concerning Dr. Glenn's wisdom in dealing with co-workers. Dr. Olley said, "I can go to Dr. Glenn, and I've gone to him, with all my facts and ducks in a row on a proposal of something we needed. Dr. Glenn would read these, sit back and say, 'Jim, I don't think it's a good time to do this. Let's hold off.' You know, he was never proved wrong. His wisdom about whether something was right or not regarding patient care always proved his decisions right, despite my facts. He was one of the most loving and caring individuals anyone could want to meet or know."

Dr. Glenn's sensitivity to the feelings of patients is revealed in a Christmas card saved from those he placed in the hands of sick patients. Above his signature he wrote: "Tonight is Christmas Eve, a time we all like to spend with our families and loved ones. We are sorry you cannot be home for the holidays but we want you to know that the nurses, doctors and dietitians and technologists will be on the job, eager to make Christmas as pleasant as possible."

During the oil shortage and energy crisis of the late 70s, Dr. Glenn (with tongue in cheek) wrote of a way to conserve energy at the hospital. "The stairs at Crawford Long are relatively easy to maintain. They have no moving parts, use no expensive electricity and require only a regular cleaning which the housekeeping department takes care of very well. One of the benefits of having stairs here at Crawford Long is that they can be used to maintain employee health. Taken in moderation, one flight up or two down the stairs provides a little bit of exercise during time otherwise spent in waiting for an elevator."

Dr. Glenn illustrates the benefits of using the stairs.

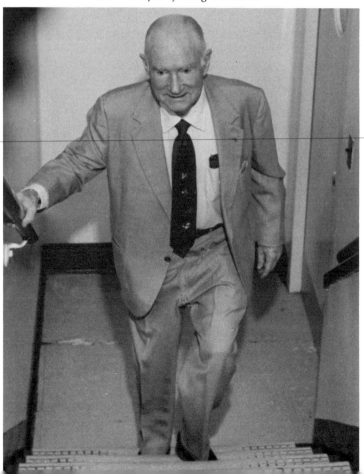

57

In another column, Dr. Glenn reminded employees of educational benefits open to them or members of their families. A full-time employee with five or more work years at Crawford Long could apply for an Emory University scholarship for a child. The chosen student would remain eligible as long as the parent was employed at the hospital and the student's grades were satisfactory. One laundry employee sent six children through school on these scholarships.

Dr. Glenn receives flu vaccine from Mrs. Evelyn McCoy, RN.

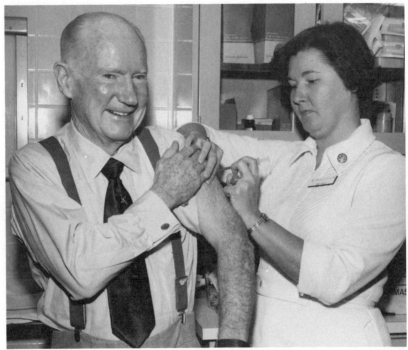

In April 1975, Dr. Glenn wrote, "Today our concerns are as much concerned with keeping people well as with restoring health. Not only is health care taking new preventative directions, but we are more and more becoming the very center of the community's health. By working to develop new methods of delivering appropriate quality care, establishing patient education programs, quality assurance, mechanisms and cost containment techniques, we are trying to make sure that when people are sick they get the right kind of care at a reasonable cost."

When a new worker joined the staff at Crawford Long, there was always Dr. Glenn's admonition: "The patient is the most important person in this institution and we must be aware that he or she is in strange surroundings, worried about himself or his family and feels an unprecedented need for compassion and understanding. We are counting on you to help make his stay as pleasant as possible."

In the later years of Dr. Glenn's tenure, some of the land surrounding the original hospital site was purchased for new additions. An Intensive Care Unit was opened in 1965 and a Coronary Care Unit in 1967.

On May 17, 1971 Dr. Glenn announced a $25 million expansion plan. Phase One, at a cost of $14 million, would place a nine-floor patient-care addition to face Peachtree Street, raising the number of beds to 520.

All this was accomplished. In a Report to the Community, Dr. Glenn replied to charges of "changes taking place and the temptation for the community hospital to try to be all things to all people." He stated that Crawford Long would concentrate on those services most urgently needed in the community and most appropriate to the Crawford Long location and resources.

Dr. Glenn emphasized that Crawford Long Hospital was in communication with other hospitals and fellow institutions, physicians in private practice, government agencies and voluntary associations. He pointed out the willingness of Crawford Long to offer services and expertise unavailable in smaller hospitals, avoiding needless duplication in selected specialties.

He cited elements which, he felt, strengthened Crawford Long's leadership position—its central location ideally situated to serve surrounding thousands of persons, an expansion program geared to better serve patients, affiliation with Emory University and the Woodruff Medical Center and its community of doctors and allied health professionals.

Added to this list was praise for a competent staff, a vibrant program and a great tradition that would work to the benefit of patients, and remarkable support from benefactors intensely interested in the welfare of the hospital and its patients.

Dr. Glenn said Crawford Long's goal of an outstanding health care system could serve as a model for the nation. "We are pressing toward that goal," he said, concluding with "What will the Crawford Long Hospital of 1980 be like? We are laying the ground work today!"

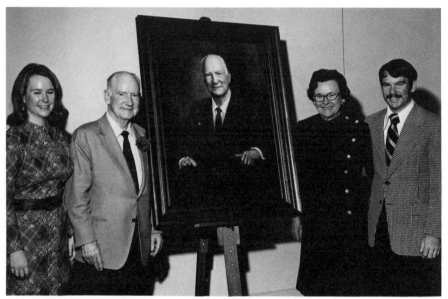

Mrs. Frances Glenn and Dr. Glenn with their children, Frances and Kearney, at the unveiling of Dr. Glenn's portrait December 15, 1972.

To mark Dr. Glenn's thirty years of service at Crawford Long, a portrait of "our good doctor" was unveiled as the climax of a December 15, 1972 Service Award Ceremony honoring him. His wife Frances and his children, Kearney and Frances, were present for the surprise portrait presentation. Mr. Daniel Barker read Nancy Yarn's poem "We Know A Man" extolling the fine qualities of the beloved physician. The last three lines of the poem summed up the regard felt for Dr. Glenn:

> For all of us love this man among men
> Our own Doctor Wadley Raoul Glenn
> He is the man!

Atlanta Mayor Maynard Jackson proclaimed February 19, 1978 as Dr. Wadley Glenn Day in Atlanta. The mayor praised Dr. Glenn for his "great perseverance, exceptional skill and tenacious will to heal and relieve the suffering of mankind for the past thirty-five years. For his capacity as Executive Director of Crawford Long Hospital of Emory University, his work as a teacher, counselor and humanitarian in the pursuit of education for many young students."

Later that same night at the Crawford Long Ball at the Chero-
kee Town Club, Dr. Glenn was presented with two bound books of
letters of tribute from his associates and friends at Crawford Long
Hospital. Henry L. Bowden, Chairman of the Emory Board of
Trustees, made the presentation.

Another recognition was presented to Dr. Glenn by Mr.
Bowden. The framed resolution commended Dr. Glenn for his active participation on Emory's Board of Trustees since 1946, and for
his outstanding achievements as an engineer, physician, teacher,
administrator, industrialist, manager and philanthropist.

The following May, Dr. Glenn and his brother Wilbur F.
Glenn received the second Woodruff Award of Dedication at a ceremony held in the Woodruff Medical Center Administration Building
at Emory. The Woodruff Award of Dedication was established in
1976 to be presented in alternate years to an individual or individuals who best exemplify the generous spirit of the award's first recipient and namesake, Robert W. Woodruff. The Glenn brothers were
chosen to receive this high award for their many years of philan-
thropic support to the Atlanta area.

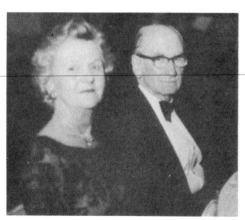

Mr. and Mrs. Wilbur F. Glenn.

When the Woodruff Award of Dedication was presented,
Robert Woodruff said, "The name of Glenn has long been identified
with the best progressive elements in business, social and professional development of Atlanta."

The keynote speaker was John Alexander McMahon, President of the American Hospital Association and Chairman of the Board of Trustees of Duke University. Emory University President James T. Laney presided at the ceremony.

The Executive Committee of the Emory University Board of Trustees, on January 2, 1985, named the operating suite of Crawford Long Hospital the Wadley R. Glenn Operating Pavilion. This action was made with the unanimous approval of the committee. On that day, it was said of Dr. Glenn, "The Wadley R. Glenn Operating Pavilion brings further distinction to the institution he helped build and so ably administered for so many years."

Mr. John D. Henry, Crawford Long Administrator, praised Dr. Glenn by saying, "Dr. Glenn was a modest man who summed up his contributions as a physician, educator and administrator as 'just part of caring for sick folks.' " Mr. Henry credited the growth of Crawford Long Hospital and its role in the Emory structure as "shaped and strengthened by Dr. Glenn at every point during his forty-five years of work and supervision there."

Dr. Glenn died on April 2, 1985 after a long battle with cancer. He was survived by his wife Frances Lewis Glenn; his daughter, Mrs. Joseph Mayson; sons, Wadley Raoul Glenn, Jr. and William Kearney Glenn; his brother, Wilbur F. Glenn; and five grandchildren.

His spirit will be a part of Crawford Long and a part of the hearts of those who worked there with him over the years. In a memorial service held that year in the Crawford Long Chapel, Chaplain Hal Jones closed his tribute to departed Crawford Long employees by saying: "Those whose names we call today died while on life's journey, but they are not forgotten. Their work at Crawford Long has helped us become who we are. Our memories of them bring tears of sadness because we miss them, but also tears of joy because of the blessing they shared. We are a better hospital, we are more giving and caring people because of how these people cared and what they gave. Our lives continue and we will move on from this place. But today the movement stops. And it stops in a moment that is ours to savor as we celebrate those who were our history, as we draw strength from those who are our heritage. Here in the peacefulness of our Chapel, and in fellowship with each other we pause, we remember, and we rediscover our hope. May God bless the memories of those whose lives have meant and will always mean so much to this community, to this hospital and to all who carry on with their work."

Dr. Glenn's name will live on in the work of those appointed to the Wadley R. Glenn Chair in Surgery at Emory University. The Glenn Chair, established in November 1984, was funded by a lead gift from the Wilbur Fisk Glenn Memorial Foundation, which was established by Thomas K. Glenn in 1947 to honor the memory of Dr. Glenn's grandfather. Dr. Charles R. Hatcher, Jr., Vice-President for Health Affairs and Director of the Robert W. Woodruff Health Sciences Center at Emory University, said: "The Glenn Chair is a fitting tribute to the surgeon who shaped and buttressed Crawford Long Hospital—Dr. Wadley Glenn."

On September 12, 1986, there was a gathering of distinguished members of the Atlanta medical community, members of the Glenn family and friends for the dedication of the Glenn Chair in Surgery. A videotape of the ceremony preserves the warmth and affection felt for Dr. Glenn by those present. There were words of praise and smiles as personal memories of Dr. Glenn were shared.

Mr. John D. Henry, Administrator and Chief Executive Officer of Crawford Long Hospital, welcomed the guests, and the Rev. Hal D. Jones, Chaplain at Crawford Long, pronounced the invocation.

Tributes were made by Mr. W. Daniel Barker, Director of Emory University Hospitals; Mr. J. W. Pinkston, Jr., Executive Director of Grady Memorial Hospital; and Dr. C. E. Holloway, former Chief of Surgery at Crawford Long Hospital. Dr. Charles R. Hatcher, Jr., presented the Chair; and Dr. Richard M. Krause, Dean of Emory University School of Medicine, accepted it.

Dr. W. Dean Warren, Chairman of the Department of Surgery, introduced Dr. John J. Coleman, III, the first holder of the Wadley R. Glenn Chair of Surgery. This is the first Emory Chair based at Crawford Long Hospital.

The video tape, "We Care," shown at the Dedication consisted of pictures and music without words. The tape showed touching scenes, commonplace in the everyday routine of hospital events, which loom large in the lives of patients. Viewers saw the gnarled hand of an elderly person clasped in the smooth hand of a nurse, patients undergoing treatment, pictures of children, and other glimpses of tender loving care. In the background, the lyrics and music of "Bridge Over Troubled Waters" told the story. It was an appropriate ballad to describe the work of Dr. Glenn.

Dr. Bishop brought the ceremony to a close with an invitation for all present to tour the new Wadley R. Glenn Operating Pavilion. Afterward, a reception was held at the Piedmont Driving Club.

Dr. Glenn's life was a bridge that stretched from the accomplishments of Crawford Long's founders to the present. His administration saw social change, awesome progress in medical science, and bold expansion with calm confidence while maintaining excellent patient care. He left a strong hospital to his successors, a challenge to keep the "Crawford Long Spirit" glowing in modern Atlanta.

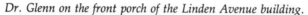

Dr. Glenn on the front porch of the Linden Avenue building.

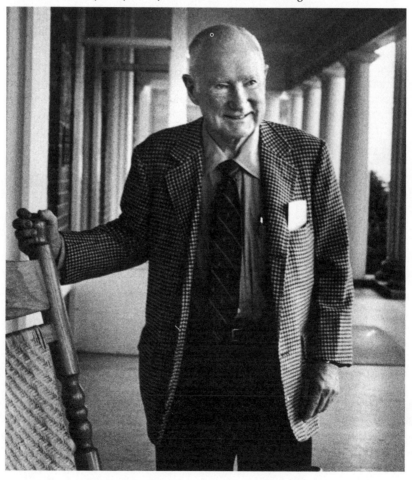

Mary G. Hart, Associate Director, Nursing Service, remembers Dr. Glenn. "This was a man who loved CWL and what it stood for. He was very visible to the staff, patients, visitors and physicians on a daily basis. He had a quick, keen sense of humor and loved life. He provided assistance to any employee in need. All you needed to do was make him aware of the need and how he could help."

In the January 1987 issue of "The Larynx," Crawford Long Administrator Mr. John D. Henry paid tribute to Dr. Glenn in an article entitled "Trademarks of Excellence—A Personal Recollection of Dr. Glenn."

He wrote: "All of us have people who have touched our lives and influenced our personal and professional development. No individual has had more influence on my life—the way I think and my desire for excellence than Dr. Wadley Glenn.

"Dr. Glenn never talked about management styles. He was a common sense manager who knew what worked. He had a gift for M.B.W.A.(management by walking around) for over forty years. He knew all employees by their first names.

"Patients were extremely important to Dr. Glenn, as individuals and also as the reason hospitals existed. He believed that if we gave high touch and high quality patient care, our patients would promote our hospital. He paid attention to all details of patient care. Impersonal care had no place in Dr. Glenn's thinking. Every patient was called by name, not room number."

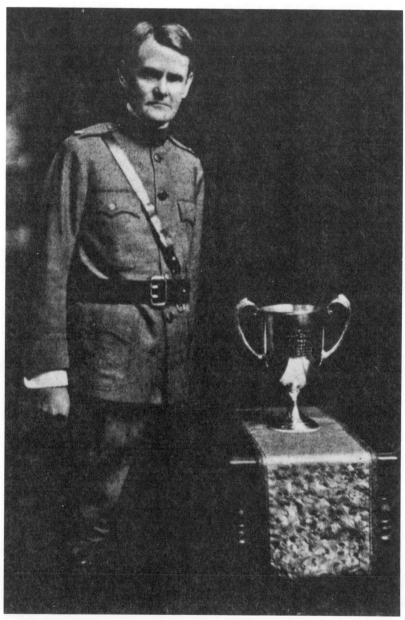

Lt.-Col. E. C. Davis "The Daddy of the Emory Unit"
(*Photo from* History of the Emory Unit)

CRAWFORD LONG UNITS
GO TO WAR

WORLD WAR I

When President Woodrow Wilson declared the United States at war with Germany and her allies in April of 1917, the call went out for doctors and nurses. Crawford Long Hospital workers joined other Americans in uniform to go to the aid of battle-weary British and French troops.

Dr. E. C. Davis, veteran of the Spanish-American War, was asked to organize Atlanta doctors. His response was prompt. He left family and home, his work at the Davis-Fischer Sanatorium, and his position as professor at Emory to become the "Daddy of the Emory Unit."

History of the Emory Unit Base Hospital #43 is a compiled oral history book of the actions and reactions of those who served in Unit #43. It is recorded there that medical technicians were so eager to enlist they stood on the bare floor of a tiny examination room at Fort McPherson Hospital awaiting their turn to be checked for duty. Once qualified, they thought they would sail for France within weeks. As it turned out, the doctors and technicians sailed that spring; the nurses followed in July.

The Army cliche, "Hurry up and wait," became reality. Thanksgiving and Christmas came and went, but on February 24, 1918, a telegram called the men to report on March 4th. On April 2, 1918, the officers of Unit #43 were ordered to Camp Gordon, Chamblee, Georgia.

A successful Atlanta newspaper campaign raised $7,000 for the Emory Unit, and a celebration was held at the Piedmont Driving Club. The $7,000 check was presented and farewell gifts of hand-knit sweaters and comfort kits were presented to volunteers by ladies of the Red Cross. Two nights later, a "farewell" service was held at Wesley Memorial Tabernacle. Methodist Bishop Warren A. Candler was the speaker.

The men spent the days waiting for action. With wry humor they trained and listened to lectures. Some of them struggled to learn French under the leadership of Mrs. Eva Woodberry, principal of Woodberry's School for Girls in Atlanta.

Atlanta women helped keep up morale with letters and packages. Mrs. W. F. Calhoun presented Dr. Davis with $50 in cash from her club. Another lady contributed an automobile to be converted into an ambulance. Mrs. John Grant offered the services of the local Red Cross Chapter to make bandages.

A dance at the Davis-Fischer Sanatorium for the men and nurses brought cheer. Then it was time for another round of goodbyes, and they boarded an outbound train described by one of the passengers as "one of Uncle Samuel's apparently cast-aside and worn-out bunch of pullman cars."

The Unit started the voyage overseas aboard the *Olympic*, escorted by a mine sweeper, but on the second day at sea it turned back. The ship's captain's announcement that one torpedo could sink the ship lent alacrity to fire and lifeboat drills, lifesaving procedures in event of an attack.

Once in the war zone, hymn sings, humorous high-jinks and pride kept morale high. When an English man-o-war steamed out from a shore-protecting smoke screen, cheers rang out. Some sang, some danced, and some prayed as a convoy of destroyers led the *Olympic* to its dock.

After two days in England, Unit #43 personnel boarded a transport to France. On the channel crossing, shared with a shipment of smelly, nervous horses, the Unit members ate meals of hard tack, corned beef and tea and sang "What's The Use Of Worrying?" and went to sleep on the planking.

They landed in France. Three days later, after a two-mile hike, they boarded a French train with berths too short for comfort. They arrived at Blois and relieved the Camp Hospital #25 personnel, to care for 416 patients.

The Blois Hospital, built in the year 854 was a convent, and then the city hall, before becoming a hospital. It charmed the Georgians even as its inconveniences were deplored.

On July 17, Major Dr. E. C. Davis was put in charge of the "first operating team." That same day a train brought 236 patients to

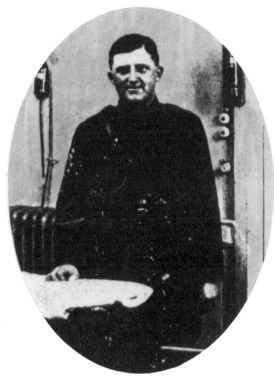

Lieutenant-Colonel Frank Kells Boland Sr. during World War I.
(Photo from History of the Emory Unit)

the Blois station. On July 22, another train arrived with 211 patients, and on August 4, a train from Chateau Thierry brought 253 men suffering from wounds, disease and the aftereffects of mustard gas.

From 1,000 patients in August the number rose to 1,825 in September. Shell-shocked casualties and German prisoners kept doctors and nurses and corpsmen working day and night. Wooden huts were thrown up to house the overflow.

Caring for gas victims was a traumatic experience. An excerpt from the Emory Unit History expresses this: "We who nursed these victims kindled anew in our hearts and minds a flame, not so much of hatred but of grim determination that they should not suffer in vain."

Battles at Chateau Thierry, St. Michiel, Belleau Woods, the Argonne and Verdun sent trainloads of shattered men to the hospital surgery unit. Regular hours were forgotten in duty to the wounded.

When an influenza epidemic struck the front, there was concern. However, death loss at Unit #43 leveled at two percent, the lowest of any hospital in France. Crawford Long people stood the test!

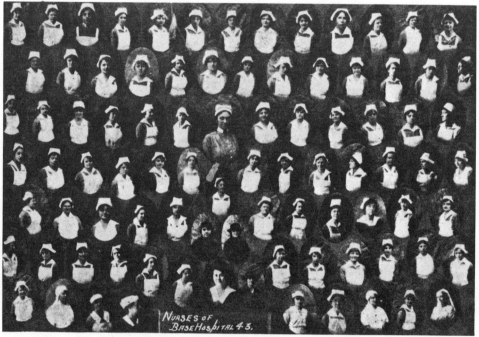

Nurses of Base Hospital No. 43. (Photo from History of the Emory Unit)

There isn't much written about the nurses who served during either of the two World Wars, and the editor of the *History of the Emory Unit* expressed regret at the paucity. It is recorded that Crawford Long Chief Nurse Caroline Dantzler was among the nurses who reported to Lakewood, New Jersey for overseas orders. While the women waited there, a nurses' flag was dedicated at Trinity Church.

On July 10, 1918, orders came for the nurses to leave at 7:30 p.m. So little time was given that one girl carried an electric iron, still warm from ironing her overcoat sleeve. A troop train took them to Montreal to a ship bound for Halifax. On July 12, they began their trip across the Atlantic Ocean. The sinking of a submarine in a battle with convoy destroyers added excitement to their voyage.

The nurses slept in their clothes and wore life belts on the crossing of the English Channel aboard an old battle-scarred hospital craft—*Guildford Castle*. During their train ride to Blois, they dined on fish, tomatoes, bread and jam, served without water.

A newspaper report by Ward Green of the Atlanta Journal, datelined Blois, France, December 19, 1918, mentions the "wonderful service of the nurses from Davis-Fischer, Wesley Memorial, St. Joseph, Grady, and other Atlanta hospitals to the war-wounded."

He wrote: "Short-handed as they were, working long hours, they went to it with a smile of cheer that has made many a dough-boy look up to them as more than angels."

A personal letter to the Atlanta Journal by a patient said: "This writer, after a slight gassing, had the misfortune to again fall ill and was sent to Base Hospital #43, in charge of the Emory Unit from Atlanta. During the year that I have been over here, I've often thought of the hospital units from the South and wondered how they would make out. I found out quickly.

"After being put out to bed, someone came in with a smile that only a woman can give and said, 'Is there anything I can do for you?' It wasn't so much the question of helping me but it was the tender way in which it was said and done that appealed to me, and there you have the spirit of your unit from Atlanta.

"Atlanta, you can well be proud of Emory Unit. And if you think you have more like it, send them along, but you'll have to go some to keep with Emory. God bless you, People of the South— From a Northern Yank, Lt. E. H. Jeffries, USA = APO N 726."

The streams of wounded continued until November 10. The Armistice, on November 11, ended the war but not the suffering. In Blois, to the amazement of the Americans, the ever-clanging bells were strangely silent. However, in the afternoon, the St. Louis Cathedral bells rang out and Allied Nations flags appeared as the streets filled with confetti-throwing, happy crowds.

A parade of Americans marched down the street to the strains of "Dixie." It was reported: "The alert attitude of every American soldier in the procession seemed to say 'That's my song.' There was no longer a north or south, east or west, but simply an America of Freedom whose sons now were treading the streets of France as comrade in arms with Allied Nations."

On Christmas Eve, the medics cheered at the reading of a

telegram from General John Pershing, their Supreme Commander. It said: "Please accept for yourself, the officers, nurses and men under your command, and patients under your care, my most cordial Christmas greetings. With appreciation of the spirit of loyalty and enthusiasm with which the personnel of your hospital has met their obligations and admiration for the unflinching fortitude with which the sick and those wounded in battle have met their misfortune. I trust that the coming year will bring to all of you happiness which you so well deserve.—PERSHING."

The wounded continued to pour into the Blois Hospital, but Unit #43 was released to go home by replacement.

After many delays, the day of departure came. Men of the Unit marched three miles to board the *Kroonland* bound for Newport News, Virginia. Dr. Henry Sauls smiled as he reported only four "cooties" [lice] were found in the contingent of 200 men of #43.

When Unit #43 was relieved after six months and eighteen days of duty in the American Expeditionary Force, it was reported that there were only 102 deaths of 9,034 patients treated; that the Unit was free of cross-infection and epidemics common during that time.

The nurses reached New York on March 12 to be greeted by cheering Red Cross, Salvation Army, YWCA and YMCA members. In Atlanta, band music, fluttering flags, relatives and friends greeted them. When Major Frank Boland appeared, they ran to shake his hand. The band played "Hail, Hail, the Gang's All Here" as they marched to meet Dr. E. C. Davis. They were honored at a dinner at Wesley Memorial Hospital on Auburn Avenue (which later became part of Emory Hospital), where Albert Dozier greeted them.

Once home, the nurses spoke of the bravery of the American soldiers under their care. One said, "We're ready to go back tomorrow if we are needed."

When the train bringing home the men of Unit #43 puffed into the yard, Dr. Davis was there to meet it. Defying orders that no one be on the tracks, he broke the line and ran to the cars. "These are my boys," he shouted. "I have worked with them and I'm going to see them right now." He was aboard and shaking hands with the men before the train came to a halt.

Tears were shed when the Emory Unit gathered for its last formation on April 2, 1919. Speeches were made, a loving cup was presented to "Lt. Col." Davis, and it was voted to form a permanent organization.

Dr. Davis was named president, Lt. Col. Frank K. Boland was vice-president, Lt. Col. Cyrus W. Strickler was 2nd vice-president, and SFC Patrick N. B. Hampton was secretary. This group met for reunion barbecues at the Davis Farm for many years to share their memories of World War I. Unit #43 became a part of history shared by doctors, nurses and corpsmen who had served at Crawford Long before the war, and many who returned there to take up work interrupted by service to their country.

WORLD WAR II

With the threat of World War II, a call came again for doctors and nurses. Crawford Long people responded again. In June 1940, the United States War Department requested assistance from Emory. A book published in 1983, *The 43rd General Hospital, World War II—The Emory Unit,* mentions the significant contributions of Dr. W. W. Strickler, Jr. and Drs. Kells and Joe Boland, sons of men who had served in WWI. By the middle of summer 1942, a full

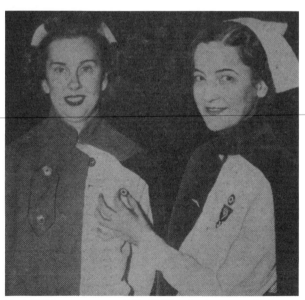

Ruth Babin, a veteran of World War I, pins a new Red Cross pin on Agnes Renfroe. Miss Renfroe, head nurse at Crawford Long, was preparing to serve in World War II. (Photo from Atlanta Journal/Constitution)

complement of officers, 100 nurses and 500 enlisted men were ready
to serve. There were people from Crawford Long in the group. The
men and women resigned from their jobs, gave up their living
quarters, made out wills, sold their cars, and said good-bye to families and friends. The Emory Unit was mobilized at Camp Livingston,
Louisiana in September 1942.

The troop trains of ancient railroad cars provided rides that
were crowded and uncomfortable. There were training sessions,
rumors of movement and maneuvers, marches and long spells of
boredom.

Christmas was merry and bright for the families who came
to Alexandria to share the holidays or for those lucky enough to go
home on leave—leave that might be the last they would enjoy until
after the war was over.

A choir was formed and ball games were organized as the
warm spring lengthened into a hot, humid, chigger-infested Louisiana summer. Nurses laughed and cried as they battled mildew in
the humid climate that left laundered clothes wet after a day of
"drying." They endured the summer's dust and shivered when fall
rain and inadequate gas heaters made their barracks anything but a
home away from home. Their fortitude did not go unnoticed. The
camp's commanding officer commended the personnel of Unit #43
for their high morale.

Emory banner of 43rd General Hospital. Left to right, Lt. Col. Ira A. Ferguson,
Second Lt. Loyce Douglas, Col. LeRoy D. Soper, C. O., First Lt. Susan W.
LaFrage, Lt. Col. R. Hugh Wood, Second Lt. Minnie O. Persons. (Photo from The
43rd General Hospital World War II)

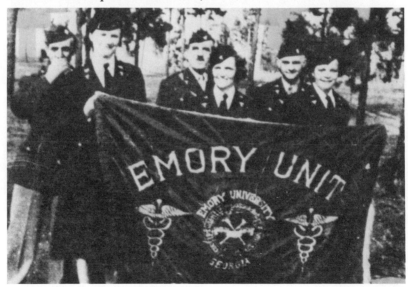

In August 1943, the Unit embarked for North Africa, their secret destination, after a sweltering forty-eight hour train ride. Their transport, the *Henry Gibbons,* was built to carry freight and 150 passengers and had been converted to carry 1,900 service people. Now it carried 2,500. It wasn't a luxury cruise. Meals were served twice a day. The food was good but was dished out in shifts to passengers who stood close together at rows of counters as they ate.

After docking in Algeria, the unit faced a three-day trip in another hot, dusty troop train with drawn shades day and night. Again, meals were eaten at counters as the passengers swayed in the rocking train.

They arrived at the 151 Station Hospital, a former French girls school, to learn that their quarters were tents furnished with canvas cots draped with mosquito nets. Nurses slept on the ground, rolled up in their bedrolls, upon arrival. They ate C or K rations. The land was arid and dusty half the year, green and muddy during the rainy season.

On October 23, 1943 the newly constructed general hospital opened with two patients. The next day, 383 patients were brought in by ambulance during a driving rain.

In the eight months that #43rd was in Oran, 8,032 patients were treated. Usually, teams worked twelve-hour duty stints from noon to midnight, midnight to noon. They often ate C rations and were without an adequate water supply.

A highlight of the Oran tour of duty was the wedding of Lt. Melba McClendon to Captain Sephus Everitt, a dentist. The war zone wedding gown, decorations and ceremony were such a success that Captain Kells Boland wanted to know who was the chief of the wedding preparations. "I've been to a lot of pretty weddings in my life but this is the prettiest one I've ever been to," he said.

An excerpt from Captain Robert Mabon's war diary, dated December 24, 1943, says: "Tonight was had a cantata—the chaplain was mainly responsible and it was very good! There were solos and a pageant and the choir was superb. All in attendance had candles and sang well. Later we had cake and cocoa. Certainly the Yuletide Spirit was not missing in our area. Today, one of the bombers around here hit Lion Mountain. There were no survivors. It has been misty and foggy as well as rainy. Tomorrow, Christmas in North Africa!!!"

On July 6, 1944 the Unit boarded a hospital ship, the *Shamrock,* bound for Naples, Italy. Here the hospital was reorganized to handle a 1,500-bed unit.

In September the hospital moved again, to Marseilles, France. From there it moved to Aix-En-Provence where more than half of the 1,500 patients were Americans. The rest were German prisoners.

At this time, the new "miracle drug" penicillin came into use saving many lives. The hospital reported treating 16,511 patients in six months.

2nd Lt. Mary Smith, a Crawford Long Nursing School graduate became part of those who served in Louisiana and then in the North African combat zone. She remembered, "It was always cold there at night, even in the summertime." From there she went into Italy with the invasion forces and on to France, where she shivered through "the coldest winter registered in 100 years. Nurses slept on canvas cots, covered up with three rough, brown army blankets piled over our bedrolls that were also the storage place for our personal items."

During her last months in the European Command, she was part of a company of eighteen nurses and twelve doctors caring for the streams of wounded being brought into a field hospital. "There were no sheets or anything," she said. "The American soldiers were laid across wooden saw horses still on the litters that brought them in. We did what we could for them and then they were evacuated by air to a general hospital further back. German prisoners were laid on the ground in aisles with hardly enough room to walk between them. Many of them were young boys of the home guard, about thirteen or fourteen years old. One of them bragged he had shot down a plane.

"We slept in our clothes," she said. "In the time we were there, we were so busy the platoons only got together a few times until after peacetime. We were devoted to the patients and their welfare," she said. "War nurses were volunteers. We were not drafted. We were dedicated because this was our choice."

First Lt. Smith, who attained her rank after five years of service, was awarded three battle stars for her service in combat zones in Africa, France and Germany. When the Korean War began, she again volunteered and served there. She later became a public health nurse.

Hospital Unit #43 returned to the United States at war's end to be inactivated at Camp Miles Standish, Massachusetts.

Veterans of World War II tell many stories of their war experiences. One is an adventure involving Dr. Kells Boland, who was assigned to accompany a detachment of rangers whose mission

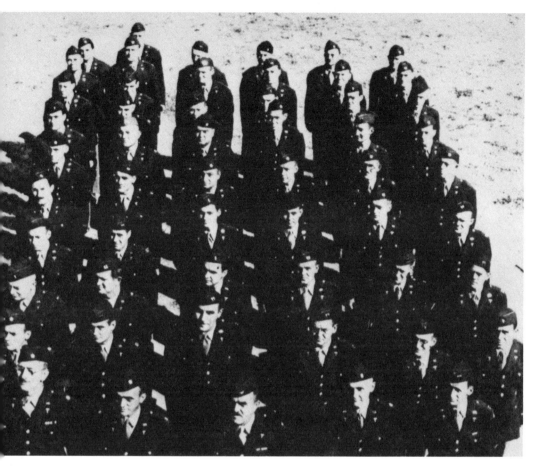

Medical, Dental and Administrative Officers at Camp Livingston, 1942

2nd/Lt. J. M. Tye 1st/Lt.	1st Lt. A. Verhoestra Capt.	Capt. J. W. Chambers Capt.	Maj. F. Parker Capt.	Maj. W. B. Bryant Chap.	Maj. H. Joiner Maj.
L. Kahn Capt.	R. Gillepsie Capt.	J. H. Boland 1st/Lt.	B. J. Hoffman Capt.	R. Andersen 1st/Lt.	S. Claiborne 1st/Lt.
S. M. Everett Capt.	H. Gibbony Maj.	H. Andrews Maj.	W. Goodyear Maj.	H. Crosswell Capt.	A. Leland Capt.
E. Rassmussen Maj.	M. K. Bailey Maj.	B. R. Burke Maj.	J. H. Harpole Maj.	E. Bosworth Capt.	C. Stone Maj.
J. M. Monfort Maj.	A. O. Lynch Capt.	J. B. Cross 1st/Lt.	C. W. Strickler Capt.	A. E. Boling Capt.	W. Trimble Capt.
G. Beck Capt.	A. E. Hauck Capt.	D. Varner 1st/Lt.	A. D. Ferguson Capt.	R. Mabon Capt.	R. Gibson Capt.
W. Funkhouser Chap.	W. B. Armstrong Capt.	F. Smith Capt.	J. H. Lange Capt.	E. B. Agnor 1st/Lt.	G. Myers 1st/Lt.
V. J. Brosnan Maj.	F. K. Boland Capt.	J. Weinberg Col.	J. Hughes Lt/Col.	J. Quinn Capt.	R. Reedy
J. D. Martin Maj.	N. Wheeler Lt/Col.	L. D. Soper	R. H. Wood	J. T. Richards	
M. Blackford	I. A. Ferguson				
File 1	File 2	File 3	File 4	File 5	File 6

Read from bottom to top beginning with File 1. (Photo from The 43rd General Hospital World War II) was to destroy several light towers hampering the landing of combat troops. Despite lack of previous training, Dr. Boland accepted the assignment. A small group of men was dropped off in rafts to paddle to an island about six hours before the time set for the invasion. After a safe landing, Major Boland's group made ready to destroy the towers.

When they were observed, enemy fire began raining down on them. With urgent speed they dug foxholes, even using the bill end of a steel helmet as a spade.

An explosion hit nearby. The soldier helping Dr. Boland was killed. A shaken Dr. Boland continued with the mission. With the beginning of the main invasion, the Germans retreated and Dr. Boland went to the 11th Evacuation Hospital to be reunited with some of the Emory Unit people stationed there.

Zola Lacretia Thomas Shanks and Bessie Henderson in 1914. Zola Thomas was the first woman anesthetist in Atlanta.

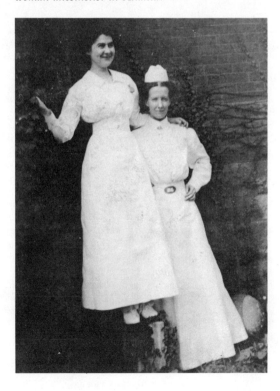

Many years later, it was discovered that Dr. Wadley Glenn, Bill Moore (the hospital's Chief Engineer), and Tom Jones (the Laundry Director) were all present on the *Missouri* when the peace treaty between the United States and Japan was signed in September of 1945. At the time, they weren't acquainted.

An interesting footnote to the history of Crawford Long's participation in World War I is the part Zola Lacretia Thomas Shanks played. Trained at the Mayo Clinic in Rochester, Minnesota, Miss Thomas came to Atlanta in 1913 to work as the chief anesthetist at Henry Grady Memorial Hospital, and was Georgia's first woman anesthetist. She later worked at Georgia Baptist Hospital before joining the Emory Unit #43 as a civilian worker.

While working near the front lines in France, she met Dr. Edgar D. Shanks. They were married in July 1919, and she retired from hospital work to raise her family. She and her husband joined to sponsor a memorial to Dr. Crawford Long in Jefferson, Georgia. She died in 1948.

Volunteers from Crawford Long took up and performed heroic (and sometimes unheralded) deeds. They endured the demands of service for their country and returned to civilian life without much fanfare. Many came back to work at Crawford Long Hospital.

A returning sailor takes wife and baby home.

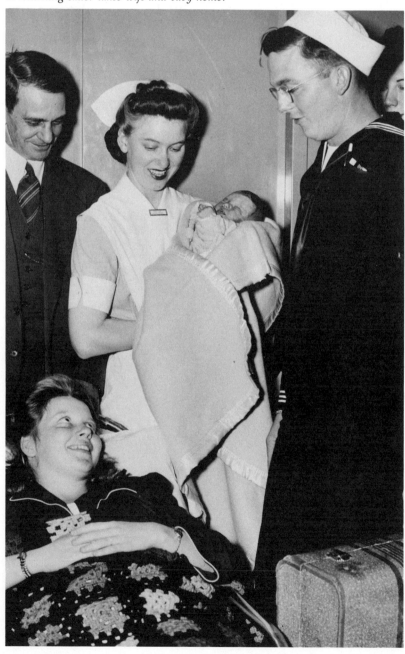

HOSPITAL EXPANSION

@rawford Long Hospital continued to grow. When the Hospital Annex opened in 1921, a newspaper article told of a new system of identifying the newborn to prevent a mixup of babies. Infants were tagged with a wrist strap and an ink footprint was made to go along with fingerprints on the chart of the new mother before the child was dressed. Then mother and child were tagged with metal disks bearing matching numbers before the newborn child was brought to the mother.

Another innovation, eliminating the annoying bell ringing to summon a nurse, was a system of blue and red call lights installed over the hall doors of patient rooms. With patient pressure on the electric button by the bed, the call room nurse was alerted immediately. Charts, instrument racks and other necessities in the call room were built especially to save lost motion.

The first two floors of the new fireproof building housed seventy-five nurses and student nurses. The laundry, dispensaries and storerooms were in the basement. The five upper stories held private rooms, wards, diet kitchens, sterilizing and medicine rooms, and offices.

A roof garden of plants, white columns, and a fountain and a sun parlor with wide windows made delightful retreats for patients and staff members on break.

In October 1921, the Davis-Fischer Sanatorium was one of seventeen Georgia hospitals on the approved list of general hospitals of one hundred beds or more by the Clinical Congress of the American College of Surgeons. This commendation meant Davis-Fischer Sanatorium met the highest standards required by an up-to-date hospital facility.

As time passed, there were other improvements in patient treatment and plans for expansion to meet increasing demands for hospital beds.

Mr. E. F. C. Fisk, the first Crawford Long Hospital Administrator, remembers the expansion work in the 1940s. "During World War II," he recalls, "we had a Cadet Nurse Training Program which the federal government helped fund. To accommodate extra people, Dr. Fischer bought two apartments and a restaurant on Prescott Street. We remodeled them to suit our needs.

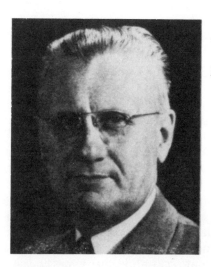

Hospital Administrator Mr. E. F. C. Fisk in a 1955 photo from The Phenap.

"At that time, two buildings were remodeled for patient use. The Pharmacy moved and new equipment was purchased for the laundry. The ground floor of the Woodruff Building was equipped for the Dietary Department.

"We purchased 17 Prescott Street for young doctors and their families. The Byron Apartment Building on West Peachtree was purchased for doctors, nurses, anesthetists, aides, people needed for emergencies.

"Old houses on the corner of Prescott and West Peachtree and on the other side of 17 Prescott were torn down to make room for a parking space."

Marion Smith Taylor, Administrative Nurse Coordinator, Newborn Nursery, entered the Crawford Long Cadet Nurse Program on a scholarship in September 1945, to graduating in September 1948.

She said, "I enjoyed all my Nursing School experiences but when I got to the Premature Nursery, I knew it was my love." She remembers that "Crawford Long had an Obstetrical Clinic open in the 1940s in which patients were admitted for prenatal visits as soon as they knew they were pregnant. They were cared for during delivery, and until the end of six weeks postpartum. The infants were also cared for during the hospitalization. No matter how short or long the time, the fee was $27.50.

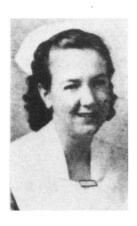

Marion Smith Taylor
in a 1947 picture
in The Phenap. *At the time,*
she was a junior in
the School of Nursing.

"The Premature Nursery was opened as a separate nursery in 1947. Before we could get started teaching the public nurses, Crawford Long and the State Health Department granted scholarships for the nurses to go to different hospitals throughout the country where there were premature nursery programs. I was fortunate enough to go to Denver, Colorado.

"At that time the Premature Nursery was instituted, there was a very large Pediatric Service with eight to ten residents, and we were having about five thousand deliveries per year. We had two newborn nurseries on fourth and fifth floors and the Premature Nursery on the Sixth Floor and Sick Newborn Nursery on the Pediatric Ward. During this time, Crawford Long did the first exchange transfusion in the Southeast."

In the early 1950s, Crawford Long also was a part of the system that saw many rural-born babies transported for care. A nurse and a resident would go to small towns and pick up babies needing special care.

"During the residency program, there was much research. I

remember the studies of Rh incompatibility and studies on B-12. During this time, with the smaller babies living, we came to see evidence of retrolental fibroplasia. . . .

"Every baby in the Premature Nursery was checked every week by ophthalmologists. There were also much research into the cause of hyaline membrane disease.

"When the suburban hospitals opened and [the number of cases in] obstetrics dropped, we didn't have as many deliveries and we didn't have as many 'preemies.'" In the latter part of 1978, Crawford Long became part of the Emory Perinatal Transport System. Fellows in Neonatology were assigned to the nursery. Crawford Long sent many nurses to Grady Memorial Hospital [to study] the theory on newer techniques in taking care of these babies.

"In the 1980s, a neonatology program was instituted and we now have a full-time neonatologist and nurse practitioners working in the nursery." (A neonatologist is a physician certified by the American Board of Pediatrics with specialized training in the care of premature infants.) The nurse practioners utilize protocols developed by the Emory Perinatal System to treat babies. They are a vital part of the care of the sick infants.

"I remember admitting patients into the recovery room when there were no beds available at Crawford Long or at other hospitals. I'm still in contact, after all these years, with people who have had babies at Crawford Long."

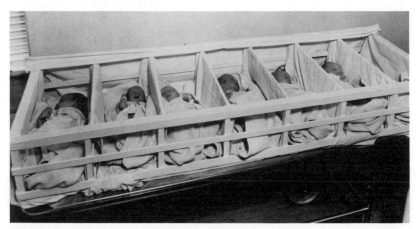

During the post-war baby boom, homemade perambulators such as this one were used to distribute newborns to their mothers.

EMILY WINSHIP WOODRUFF MATERNITY CENTER

When the Emily Winship Woodruff Maternity Center opened its doors in January 1945, fifty-five bassinets awaited newborns in triple-filtered and washed air. There were nine labor rooms and four green-tiled delivery rooms. Every precaution was taken to protect well babies from those who might be ill.

In the 40s, it was rare for a husband to be present at the birth of his child. When one husband demanded to be present, newspapers across the United States carried the story of a young Californian who chained himself to his laboring wife with handcuffs and secured the chains with padlocks. He was allowed to witness the birth.

Crawford Long doctors, in agreement with doctors in other Atlanta hospitals, did not allow the fathers in the delivery room because they believed the fathers "couldn't stand it." They thought fathers would get in the way and that the requirement for extra sterile gowns would add to the laundry load. Nurses agreed with

Two fathers "relax" in the reclining room.

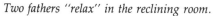

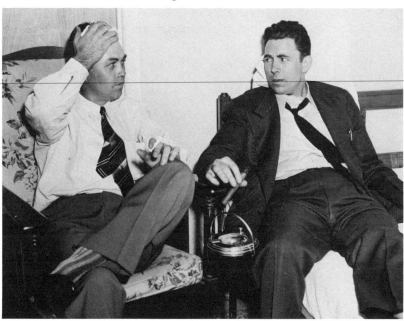

the physicians, so most husbands paced the floor, smoked, or drank coffee and soft drinks.

Crawford Long provided a "reclining room" so the floor pacers could try to relax and perhaps even sleep briefly as they waited out their wives in labor and delivery. Dr. Fischer, with his ever ready humor, commented, "We have never lost a father yet, but we have come dangerously nigh to it. This father's room is an added precaution."

In March of 1943, Dr. Fischer wrote to actress Greer Garson to tell her how much he was impressed by the movie, "Blossoms In The Dust." He explained he was so moved by her portrayal of the true story of Mrs. Gladden's Texas effort to have the word "illegitimate" removed from birth certificates there that he used his influence to have Bill #459 presented to the sitting Legislature. This bill became a Georgia law. Thereafter "illegitimate" was no longer used on a birth certificate.

In his letter, Dr. Fischer pointed out that at Crawford Long Hospital, in 1942 and until March of 1943, of 2126 deliveries, not one mother was lost! The national average at that time was seven moth-

Personnel and visitors enter the newly opened
Emily Winship Woodruff Maternity Center in 1945.

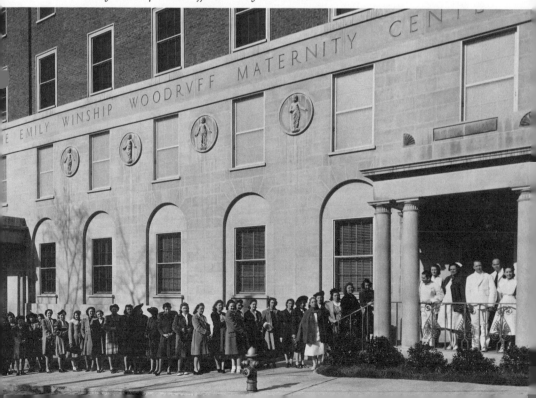

ers per thousand. Greer Garson congratulated him on his accomplishments in a reply.

Another maternity story involves Dorothy Nix, Executive Director of the DeKalb Historical Society. Thirty years ago, her husband was told she didn't have much chance of surviving. Mrs. Nix said, "If I had not been in Crawford Long, I never would have made it."

She came into the hospital in distress. Her doctor, who was shopping that December 10, 1950, was hastily summoned. He found Mrs. Nix in shock. A Caesarian section was immediately ordered, and the Rh Negative blood that was on hand for the baby, in case it was needed, was used to save the mother's life.

Back in her room and very ill, Mrs. Nix said, "The word 'Life' from the Life of Georgia Building sign nearby was visible from my bed. That word 'Life' was like a good omen to me," she said, "It gave me strength."

Her son, after birth, spent a short time in a machine called an "Airlock." Mrs. Nix said, "I believe Crawford Long was the only place that had an Airlock, something like a miniature iron lung."

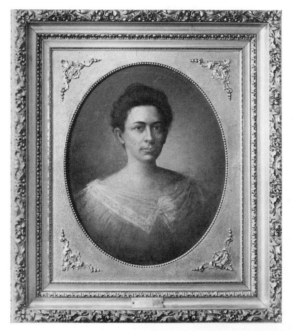

Mrs. Cora Best Taylor Williams. Her portrait and that of her husband hang in the administration office of the Jesse Parker Williams Pavilion in Crawford Long Hospital.

Jesse Parker Williams

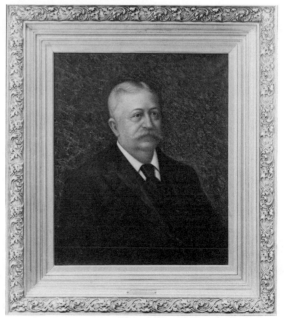

JESSE PARKER WILLIAMS STORY

𝒥esse Parker Williams Hospital, an independent medical unit within the walls of Crawford Long Hospital, is located on the first floor of the building on Peachtree Street. It serves as an independent hospital, just as it has since it was chartered in 1930.

Cora Best Taylor Williams was the wife of Jesse Parker Williams, a graduate of the University of Virginia, who came to Georgia after service in the Confederate Army during the Civil War. He made a fortune in lumber, naval stores, and railroad holdings in the Georgia, Florida, and Alabama Railroad. When he died in 1913, Mrs. Williams took over the management of his business.

Cora Williams was known for her beauty and her sharp mind for business. She maintained homes in Lanark, Florida, in Statesboro, Georgia, and in Atlanta, and wisely conducted her late husband's business affairs. She became president of the Georgia, Florida, and Alabama Railroad, the only woman railroad president in the world.

She never lost sight of the fact her fortune was the result of her husband's initiative and hard work. She also remembered long days of invalidism due to illness when she was a child, a memory that made her determined to help alleviate the suffering and panic of such illness in a family without money and nowhere to turn for help.

Before her death in 1924 after a long bout with cancer, she decided to provide hospitalization and medical care for those women and children whose private funds had been exhausted. Under the terms of her will, a hospital building was to be constructed on a suitable Georgia site. Five Georgians were to be appointed trustees to administer the funds, operate the hospital and pay whatever part was necessary to meet the medical expenses of women, female children, and male children under twelve years of age. The institution would be named the Jesse Parker Williams Hospital as a tribute to her husband.

It was 1940 before her complicated estate was finally settled, although the prospective hospital's charter was accepted by the trustees in June of 1930. Setbacks came when the estate administrator's widow, Mrs. John Lord Nisbet, brought suit for fees she felt Mrs. Williams had promised her husband. After trial and appeal, the question was settled and work proceeded.

After checking into several locations in Atlanta, the trustees decided to use the site of Mrs. Williams' home at 542 Peachtree Street, on the same block as Crawford Long Hospital. The Jesse Parker Williams Hospital contracted with Crawford Long for all intern and nursing care, for the use of the operating rooms, X-ray, laboratory services, meals, and laundry.

A small modern hospital with 63 beds, waiting rooms and a lobby, private rooms and wards was built. More patients could be treated with less funds because of the arrangement with Crawford Long.

The first patient stayed 6 days. The bill was $24.

When Crawford Long's Peachtree Building was planned, the contract continued. The Jesse Parker Williams Hospital trustees conveyed the title to the land and hospital building plus $500,000 in cash to Crawford Long Hospital in exchange for an equity in the new hospital plant equivalent to one patient floor of approximately equal size and patient capacity to the facilities formerly owned by Jesse Parker Williams Hospital to operate as a separate and independent hospital.

Crawford Long continues to provide services to Jesse Parker Williams Pavilion of Crawford Long Memorial Hospital as was agreed. The Williams Hospital occupies the entire first patient floor of the Peachtree Building, and houses 50 pediatric, surgical, and medical patient beds.

Part of the Peachtree Building encompasses the Peachtree frontage of the original Jesse Parker Williams Hospital. The rear section has been incorporated into Crawford Long and is used by the Physical Therapy and Engineering Departments.

The Joint Commission on Accreditation of Hospitals found this "hospital within a hospital" arrangement unique. After checking and rechecking, they wrote up their findings and placed the

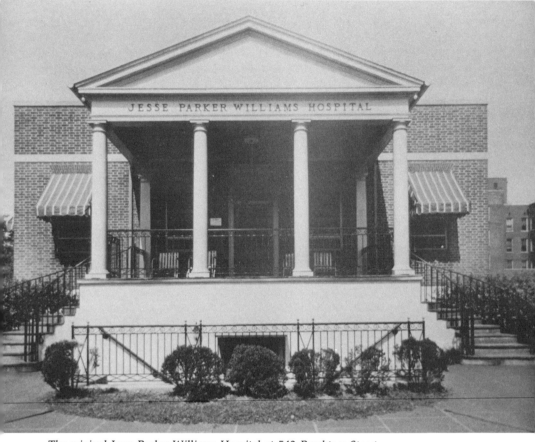

The original Jesse Parker Williams Hospital at 542 Peachtree Street.

outline and their approval in permanent files for the use of future investigators.

Mrs. Betty Lee, Secretary-Treasurer of the Jesse Parker Williams Board of Trustees, said she could understand the problem in comprehending the Williams-Crawford Long setup. Subsequent inspections revealed surprise at the successful arrangement Mrs. Lee says "has worked out beautifully through the years, with Crawford Long doing everything in its power to make the patients of Jesse Parker Williams Hospital have outstanding medical care.

"Since the hospital first opened, there have been four administrators. Mrs. Ruth Sheafe was first. When she retired, Mrs.

Janet Lorenz took her place. After Mrs. Lorenz retired (about the same time we came under the new hospital setup in our beautiful new building), Miss Mamie Lowe Hubbard took over. Upon her retirement, Mrs. Freda Moss became Administrator."

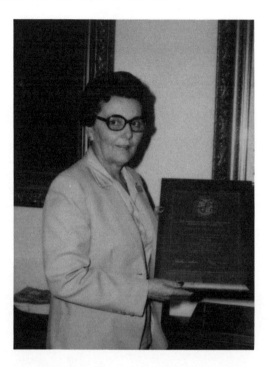

Freda Moss, Jesse Parker Williams Hospital Administrator, holds a plaque presented by the American Hospital Association. The plaque recognizes Jesse Parker Williams Hospital's fifty years as a member of the Association.

Two other programs were implemented by the trustees under the leadership of William C. Wardlaw, Jr.

One program established the Jesse Parker Williams Garden Wing of the A. G. Rhodes Home. The Garden Wing accommodates 35 women, all nursing care patients. General hospital services are furnished by the Rhodes Home, and payment for qualified patients' care is assisted by Jesse Parker Williams.

The Jesse Parker Williams Pavilion fills the 7th floor of the Budd Terrace in Wesley Homes, caring for 43 qualified patients under agreement with Wesley Homes. Here food, laundry, and occupational therapy are furnished by Wesley Homes.

Mr. and Mrs. Williams are buried in Westview Cemetery where their resting place is marked by a monument executed by the famous sculptor, Daniel French.

TRUSTEES, JESSE PARKER WILLIAMS HOSPITAL, INC.

May 27, 1987

Name	Years of Service
Dudley Cowles	1929-1937
Clark Howell, Jr.	1929-1966
Neal Meier	1929-1936
C. F. Palmer	1929-1940
Philip Weltner	1929-1932 & 2/23/39 to 10/9/39
John Lord Nisbet	1932-1938
W. E. Mitchell	1936-1960
W. E. Harrington	1937-1945
Thomas K. Glenn	1940-1945
R. B. Wilby	1940-1960
Charles H. Jagels	1945-1960 & 1965-1977
A. Steve Clay	1945
N. Baxter Maddox	1945-1976
Robert F. Adamson	1960-1976
William C. Wardlaw	1960-1983
James M. Sibley	1966-present
Henry T. Collinsworth	1976-present
Edward P. Gould	1976-present
J. Robin Harris	1977-present
John H. Weitnauer, Jr.	1984-present

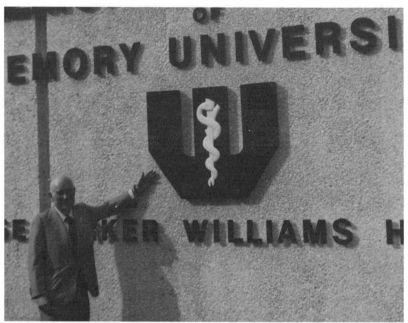

Dr. Glenn with the new "W" logo of the Woodruff Health Sciences Center.

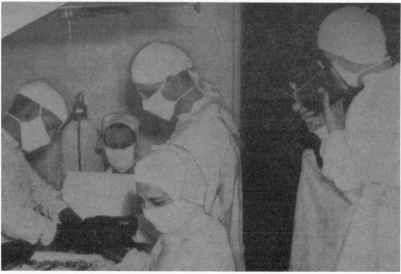

In this picture from The Atlanta Journal, March 28, 1937, Miss Alice R. Thompson is shown photographing an operation at Crawford Long.

IMPORTANT FIRSTS

@rawford Long Hospital, from its beginning, has been an innovator in medical care. Its list of "firsts" is long and impressive. Some of these are small but important accomplishments; others are spectacular breakthroughs in medicine. Each has contributed to Crawford Long's outstanding reputation among teaching hospitals.

Behind each is a person who fostered a new idea from conception to realization, working alone or with a team, to improve accepted medical treatment procedures. Like Crawford Long, Dr. Fischer and Dr. Davis, they dared to make their dreams come true.

EARLY VIDEO INSTRUCTION

In the spring of 1937, Alice Thompson, Superintendent of Nurses, made motion pictures of complicated operations for the instruction of student nurses and interns. The surgery was performed by surgeon-professors of medical schools.

Miss Thompson said then the doctors were so intent on their work they forgot they were being filmed.

AIR CONDITIONING A NEW COMFORT

On August 8, 1939, a woman from East Point delivered her son in the air-conditioned Crawford Long maternity ward, the first air-conditioned maternity ward in the Southeast. At that time, there was more than passing interest in "the new science of air conditioning" that allowed a 70 degree temperature in the birthing room while the thermometer outside crept upward in the hot Georgia sun.

TRIPLETS SURVIVE

In 1939 the Allen triplets, the first trio ever to survive Caesarian delivery in the United States, were born at Crawford Long Hospital under the watchful care of Dr. Linton Smith and Dr. Don Cathcart. The two little boys and their sister lived in Room 301-B until they were twenty months old, since their mother had died at their birth. The nursery workers cared for them with extra doses of TLC. One of the nursery workers became the triplets' stepmother a few years later when she and their father married.

By the time Crawford Long celebrated its Fiftieth Anniversary in 1961, the triplets had graduated from high school and were doing well. The three said they didn't remember being the pets of the staff.

Estelle Henderson, RN, said at the close of her thirty-fifth year of duty, "If you want to know the event I remember most about the past thirty-five years, it would be the birth of the triplets in 1939. How I cried when we lost their mother."

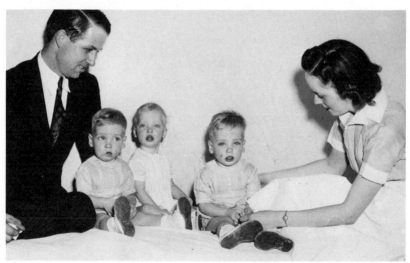

Mr. Fred Allen with his triplets. This photo was taken in May 1941, when Ralph, Ruby, and Robert were two years old.

RECOVERY ROOM MEETS A NEED

Georgia Belle Hearn Martin, RN, was part of the team that established the first hospital recovery room in the Atlanta area, a novel idea in 1944. Now an accepted part of hospital procedure everywhere, it's difficult to imagine efficient post-operative care without it. Prior to World War II, post-operative patients were sent to their original rooms, attended by a nurse and an anesthetist, until they were sufficiently recovered to be left to floor nursing or family member care.

With the wartime nursing shortage, there simply were not enough people to go around, and since Dr. Glenn was away serving in the Navy, his suite of offices was used as the first recovery room. Beds were placed in his reception room, and his paneled office became the sleeping quarters for anesthetists. Another room became an isolation spot for possibly infectious patients.

DR. DOWMAN'S DESIGN

On January 5, 1947, Dr. Charles Dowman used hypothermia to successfully perform neurosurgery on a patient from Texas. Although there had been one or two cases of heart surgery in which the principle of hypothermia (the lowering of body temperature below 98.6) had been used, this was its first use in neurosurgery.

Dr. Dowman designed a body trough which was built especially for this operation. Assisting Dr. Dowman was cardiologist, Dr. Manuel Cooper, and two anesthetists, Dr. Sotolongo and Dr. Geerkin.

DAY NURSERY CARE FOR NURSES' CHILDREN

The Crawford Long Day Nursery, the first in Atlanta to be operated for hospital personnel, was the 1947 forerunner of now-common care centers for employees' children. It was set up by Georgia Belle Hearn Martin.

Mrs. Martin asked a former classmate to come back to work in the Nursing Service, only to be told she could not because she had no one to care for her child. Mrs. Martin asked her if such care could be provided, would she give an affirmative reply. The answer was "Yes." The nursery was opened on the 6th floor of the C

Building, which was not in use.

It wasn't long before other nurses responded, and Mrs. Martin, pleased with the success, decided to get some little publicity to stimulate nursing recruitment.

The first newspaper article brought unforeseen results! A representative of the City Health Department called to see if the nursery had a license—a detail never thought of by Mrs. Martin in her enthusiasm for a solution to a worrisome problem. Investigation of the Day Nursery found it well within the rules and regulations. By 1961, it was operating on a sixteen-hour-a-day schedule caring for fifty-one children of working graduate nurses.

The Day Care Center became a model for such establishments across the State of Georgia and often was referred to by the State Licensing people as an excellent example of a good child care program. It was closed in 1979. Miss Pope, Assistant Administrator for Nursing Service, said, "Unfortunately, the cost of operating such an outstanding nursery which included a kindergarten caused us finally to close the nursery. We felt we could no longer justify the big outlay of investment with no great return. It was, however, a model which served us for many years."

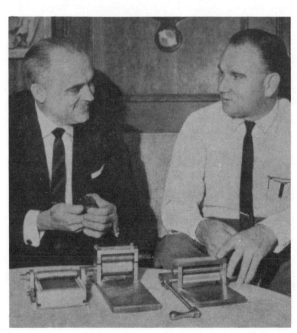

W. H. Bradley and Dr. J. C. Tanner look over models of the Meshgraft Dermatome. Mr. Bradley served as a technical advisor to the project. (Photo from the Atlanta Journal/ Constitution).

FIRST BLOOD BANK AND RH TRANSFUSION

In 1947, Crawford Long established the first blood bank in Atlanta with complete Rh testing. An emergency donor list, including three hundred staff members, was set in place. At this time, Crawford Long Hospital was one of two Atlanta hospitals capable of operating independently of the American Red Cross.

In 1948, Crawford Long was the scene of the first blood transfusion performed on an Rh baby.

FIRST LONG BED

A big relief for tall patients was the 1961 purchase of a ninety-inch long bed to accommodate the taller-than-average person. This longest bed on the market was the first such stretch comfort brought into use in the Southeast.

MESHGRAFT DERMATOME

It has been called "a new miracle in skin grafting," and Crawford Long had a part in it with Dr. James C. Tanner, Jr. The time was 1964. The miracle was the restoration of live skin to a charred area of a badly burned patient.

Dr. Tanner's inspiration for this treatment came to him as he broiled on the backyard grill and noticed the pattern of the grilling rack. It was made of a piece of metal cut and stretched out to almost double its length, forming a lattice pattern with diamond-shaped openings. He wondered if pieces of human skin could be gently stretched out in a similar diamond pattern that could then be grafted over a burned area.

He enlisted the help of W. H. Bradley, who manufactured tiny steel blades used to make perforations in paper products, to make a similar tool to cut delicate slits in a length of a patient's self-donated skin.

Dr. Jacque Vandeput, a resident in plastic surgery at Crawford Long, worked with Dr. Tanner. Dr. James F. Olley did the microscope experimental work. Dr. Charles C. Rife lent his animal hospital facilities for procedure practice. Dr. H. Harlan Stone, the assistant professor in the Surgery Department of Emory School of Medicine, was also a part of the team. His case histories and photographs form an important part of the records. The research was funded by Dr. Tanner and his associates. The procedure is done with a light touch. The fragile skin is rolled and sliced into a skin ribbon mesh in a carefully monitored process and grafted. The skin, first tissue-paper thin, soon strengthens, begins to seal in vital body fluids, and keeps out infections. This process called a mesh graft, has reduced the mortality of persons with major burns.

Other Crawford Long doctors who, early on, used the Meshgraft Dermatome were Dr. John R. Lewis and Dr. J. Hagen Baskin. Doctors all over the world now use this treatment to heal the wounds of burn victims.

Dr. Tanner received the Southern Medical Association Distinguished Service Award for 1985 at the President's Doctor's Day Award luncheon on November 18. This was held at the SMA's 79th Annual Scientific Assembly in Orlando, Florida. He was cited for his lifetime devotion to surgery, research and improved care of burn patients, including his years of research in the production of the skin mesh graft technique and equipment.

TANNER-VANDEPUT PRIZE

Dr. J. C. Tanner continued to study ways to improve the care of burn patients. His own research, perfecting of techniques and new procedures, was accomplished without grants or financial help, but Dr. Tanner wanted to encourage young doctors and scientists in their studies by giving them a monetary boost. In 1984, he decided to establish the Tanner-Vandeput Prize For Burn Research.

The first person to receive the award was Ian Alan Holder, Ph.D., Director of the Department of Microbiology at the Shriner's Burn Institute in Cincinnati, Ohio.

The cash award was presented to Dr. Holder late in 1985 at a meeting of the Quadrennial Congress of the International Society for Burn Injuries held in Melbourne, Australia. Dr. Holder's research involves developing new treatments against specific infection, the leading cause of death in burn patients.

200 MILLIONTH AMERICAN

The birth of Robert Ken Woo, Jr. at Crawford Long made world news: His was the 200 millionth American birth noted by the

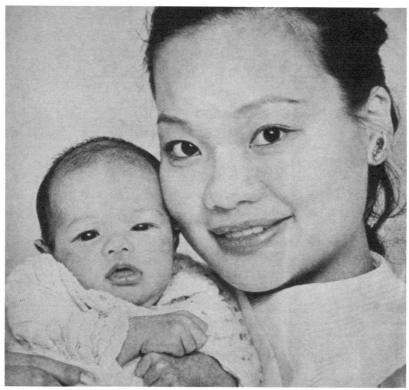

Robert Ken Woo Jr., pictured here with his mother Sally Woo,
attained instant fame when he was born in Crawford Long November 20, 1967.
He is the 200-millionth American.

Census Bureau population clock.

With Master Woo's first cry, there was applause in Washington, D.C. where President and Mrs. Lyndon Johnson awaited the birthday of the 200 millionth citizen. Dr. C. S. Glisson, Jr. declared the youngster a normal healthy male child, born at 11:03 a.m. on November 10, 1967.

His mother, Sally Woo, was born in China but left there as a child when her family fled communism. His father, Robert, is a native-born American of Chinese-American parents. Both parents are graduates of Georgia Tech.

Robert Ken Woo, Jr. was featured in a five-page spread in Life magazine on Dec. 1, 1967, as the infant who "arrived right on the spot." He was pictured with other babies who almost made the statistic as the President congratulated the 200 millionth American.

Mary Shaw, RN, who cared for Bobby Woo at birth, was delighted to learn that this celebrated boomer was, at seventeen, again in the news. Named Georgia's 1985 STAR student and Presidential Scholar, Bobby also was a finalist in the National Merit Scholarship Program. He was president of the senior class at Henderson High School in Decatur, Georgia and editor of the school's literary magazine. He was also named the varsity soccer team's most valuable player. He scored 1,540 out of a possible 1,600 on the Scholastic Aptitude Test.

Honored at the Georgia Business Council's Student/Teacher Achievement Recognition banquet, Bobby Woo was again accorded presidential recognition when a telegram of congratulations from President and Mrs. Reagan was read. Governor Joe Frank Harris spoke at the dinner honoring the state's ten Student/Teacher Achievement finalists. Selma Levy, Bobby Woo's English teacher and his choice as STAR Teacher of the Year, praised him for his humility and patience. She said, "He never makes it obvious to anyone that he is bright and capable."

His mother told of the thrill experienced by the whole Woo family when they met President Reagan and Georgia Senator Mack Mattingly at the White House where Bobby and other Presidential Scholars were congratulated on their achievements.

In the summer of 1986, Bobby completed an internship in the United States Congress. He has attended Harvard University, and his mother says he "might pursue law as a career."

The Woo's three other children, Angie, Cindy and David were also born at Crawford Long Hospital.

Life magazine remembered Bobby Woo's birth by sending him a boundcopy of its 50th anniversary issue.

QUADRUPLETS BORN

When Dr. A. C. Richardson learned from x-rays that one of his patients was carrying four infants, he made plans.

When the woman came in for delivery two-and-a-half weeks early, work was begun immediately to provide a special nursery and a room where isolettes especially purchased for the expected babies waited.

The smallest of the quadruplets born November 5, 1969 died,

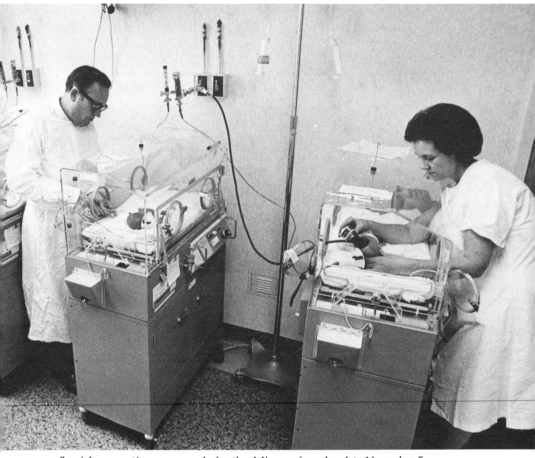

Special preparations were made for the delivery of quadruplets November 5, 1969. (Photo from the Atlanta Journal/Constitution)

but the three male survivors flourished under the watchful care of nursery personnel.

A letter to Mr. Dan Barker expressed the gratitude of the young parents. Part of it said: "We find it hard to convey just how we feel about the generosity afforded us by Crawford Long Memorial Hospital.

"Thank you so very much for all the special preparations made and the special equipment secured just for our 'special delivery.' "

ENVIRONMENTAL HEALTH

Crawford Long was the first Metro Atlanta hospital to establish an Environmental Health Department. The purpose of this department, established in 1970, was to make the hospital as safe as possible for patients, medical staff and personnel.

Dr. H. B. Stillerman, an internal medicine physician for twenty years and consultant in bacteriology at Crawford Long, with the assistance of his wife, Marguerite, a registered nurse, headed this unit. Their job was to locate sources of infections and carriers of diseases like staph, salmonella and tuberculosis. Spot checks of kitchen, operating rooms and laundry equipment would evaluate problem areas.

In August of 1973, Dr. and Mrs. Stillerman were featured in the "Larynx." They also wrote a paper for *Hospital* Magazine dealing with how to set up an environmental surveillance program. "This," Dr. Stillerman said, "was medical detective work to pinpoint sources of infection and so provide the best possible environmental health for patients and employees."

The Stillermans were also involved in teaching and research including lectures to groups of nurses and making rounds with physicians. He also conducted an infection control seminar at Georgia State University. Dr. and Mrs. Stillerman were members of a team that developed and tested "unit tube feeding." Mrs. Stillerman worked with other infection control nurses in the then new Control Association of Greater Atlanta.

INFORMATION

Sara Quillian started the Information Desk she manned for twenty-five years. When her husband, Dr. Andrew F. Quillian, died in his forties and her two daughters married, Mrs. Quillian decided she needed "something to do."

"Then," she said, "my good friend, Macie Stephens, asked me to start an Information Desk. The hospital has meant a good deal to me."

PREMATURE CARE MATURES

"Crawford Long had the first Premature Nursery in the Atlanta area," said Marion Taylor, head nurse in the 5-C Nursery. It opened in May 1972.

Fathers can visit the mother and child. "He can put on a mask and gown and stay with the mother at feeding time," Mrs. Taylor said. "But when the baby is premature, the feeding is different. As the baby matures, we let the parents help with it so they will know how to do it when they take Baby home. We don't just throw the family and baby out. We help get them ready for the new family member."

Mrs. Taylor had praise for Margaret Green, another Crawford Long graduate, and her work in the Nursery. These nurses said that even after all these years with babies, they still spoil the "preemies" and sick infants, who sometimes spend weeks in the Nursery. "I'm afraid the ones who stay a while are spoiled by us before they go home," said Mrs. Taylor with a smile.

A graduate of the Crawford Long School of Nursing, Mrs. Taylor said, "I've lived more than half my life at this hospital. It is my second home."

SMOOTH AS SILK MOVE

With the completion of the Patient Care Tower on October 1, 1973, the task of moving patients from the older units to the sparkling new rooms began.

Mrs. Ina Hooker, a 1934 alumna of the Crawford Long Nursing School, was the first patient transferred to the Coronary Unit. Shortly after she went back home, she reported the move as "smooth as silk."

A world of work, planning and coordination was necessary for the patient transfers. In early October, hospital personnel began countless trips from the old to the new facilities. Floor by floor, patients, young and old, critically ill and recovering, had to be moved, with preparations to meet any emergency carefully mapped out ahead of time.

Patients are grouped by floors according to disease types; for example, all cardiology patients were placed on one floor. This necessitated a new system for the nursing staff; they were grouped to work by clinical specialties. To treat acute illnesses, thirty-six beds were set aside for intensive care. Patients with cardiac, renal, respiratory and surgical problems would be cared for in separate units, each with the expertise and equipment geared for their particular needs.

There were other improvements as well. Heart attack victims' rides to the hospital can be monitored by special ambulance equipment that keeps them in contact with the Emergency Room staff. A coronary care waiting room with contour chairs encourages relatives to catch a few winks of sleep as they await news of their loved ones' progress.

To cut down on dust and maintenance, window blinds were sealed between panes of glass. The windows pivot for easier washing. Machines sweep, wash, dry and wax terrazzo floors in one step. Information is kept for instantaneous retrieval by computer.

The tower facilities help Crawford Long offer the best care available to the community at an economical cost.

FIRST OPEN HEART SURGERY AT CRAWFORD LONG

Open heart surgery was performed at Crawford Long Hospital for the first time on November 20, 1974 by a surgical team that included Dr. Joseph M. Craver, Dr. Joseph I. Miller, Jr., and Dr. Charles R. Hatcher, Jr. By the second week in January 1975, open heart surgery was performed on a regular basis at the Carlyle Fraser Heart Center Division of Crawford Long.

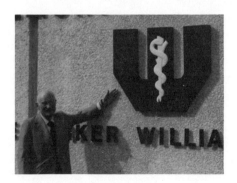

A NEW SIGN

The first exterior sign displaying the now familiar "W" logo of the Woodruff Health Sciences Center was installed on the Peachtree Building of Crawford Long on November 5, 1975. The caduceus on the logo is the symbol of medicine and consists of the staff of Aesculapius (the Greek god of medicine) about which a single serpent is coiled. (Ancient doctors wore a serpent bracelet as a mark of their profession.)

The Woodruff Medical Center was created on April 21, 1966, by a resolution of the Board of Trustees of Emory University. It was redesignated the Woodruff Health Sciences Center in 1985.

A FIRST FOR MR. BARKER

W. Daniel Barker was elected Chairman-Elect Designate of the American Hospital Association August 30, 1977. His election to this high office in the Association was the first in the State of Georgia and the Georgia Hospital Association.

A PRESIDENT VISITS CRAWFORD LONG

Sarah Rosemary Carter, first granddaughter of President Jimmy Carter, was born at Crawford Long Hospital on December 19, 1978. Sarah is the president's third grandchild. The president rode in a motorcade from Dobbins Air Force Base to Crawford Long Hospital where he and Mrs.Carter admired the newest family member.

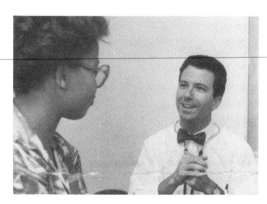

Dr. James Braude uses sign language to communicate with his deaf filing secretary, Cheryl Morgan.

WORD OF HAND

Dr. James Braude of Crawford Long Hospital is believed to be the only internist in the United States who is fluent in signing—communicating with the deaf by use of Finger Spelling, American

Sign Language or Signing Exact English (SES). He decided to learn this communication skill when he had difficulty understanding a deaf woman suffering a heart attack. He hired two instructors to teach him sign language, and he took courses, read books, and hired a deaf woman as his filing secretary to help him acquire what he calls "word of hand" to better serve deaf patients.

Dr. Braude usually speaks and signs at the same time for the benefit of patients who can read lips. He also has a special phone system that allows deaf patients to make appointments by way of a telephone digital display.

The woman whose heart attack introduced Dr. Braude to the world of the deaf survived and is still his patient. "The big difference now," he says, "is that we can talk. I speak her language."

ALL BEADS AREN'T JEWELRY

Dr. George Cierney III is a pioneer in the use of reconstructive surgery to save infected bone from amputation. For this, he uses beads—antibiotic beads.

Dr. Cierney explains "When you're planning to reconstruct an infected bone you face a conceptual problem—you have to think in 3-D.

"You have to remove the infected portion of the bone, replace it with living tissue. The big challenge is to find enough biological material to replace the defect. The antibiotic beads give you time to stage the procedure—to cure the infection, and then you begin to reconstruct the bone—rather than doing everything at once. The beads don't change what we do, they change when we do it."

Before 1986, the only treatment for bone infection was amputation. Dr. Cierney's pioneer technique is based on cancer reconstruction.

Dr. Cierney is today one of about five surgeons in the United States reconstructing bones. He has a success rate of 96%.

A PEACHTREE STREET

Crawford Long Hospital's official address is now 550 Peachtree Street, N.E., rather than at 35 Linden Avenue. But the original entrance Between the Peachtrees, so dear to many Atlantans, stands as a reminder of the beginnings of the Crawford Long Hospital complex, now covering four city blocks.

John D. Henry, Hospital Administrator, says the change of address makes it easier for patients and visitors to find the hospital. "Most everyone knows where Peachtree is," he said. "But very few people know where Prescott Street and Linden Avenue are located. As Atlanta has grown, so must Crawford Long grow. Many of our former patients and publics we have taken care of so well in the past are no longer around. We need to make this change to have better street recognition and to assist our current patients and guests in finding the hospital."

THERAPEUTIC GASTROINTESTINAL WORK

Crawford Long is a pioneer in therapeutic gastrointestinal laser endoscopy in the Southeastern United States. In May of 1980, a YAG Laser Photoagulator began operation. With this equipment, physicians can locate directly and accurately the source of any bleeding or abnormal growth and then directly aim the laser beam at the lesion. The Crawford Long YAG Laser uses a two channel endoscope developed to the specifications of Dr. R. Carter Davis, Jr. who services as GID Medical Director.

Dr. R. Carter Davis, Jr. has followed his grandfather, Dr. E. C. Davis, and his father, Dr. R. Carter Davis, Sr. in his choice of a career. A graduate of the Emory University School of Medicine, he did post-graduate work at Cornell University Medical Center, at

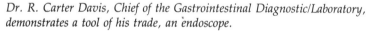

Dr. R. Carter Davis, Chief of the Gastrointestinal Diagnostic/Laboratory, demonstrates a tool of his trade, an endoscope.

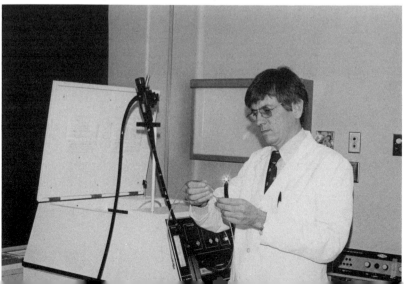

Mainz University Medical School, Germany and at the University of Wisconsin where he studied with the famous Dr. John Morrisey. He came to Crawford Long in the fall of 1972, bringing his special fiber-optic endoscopic instruments such as duodenscopes, colonoscopes, and special gastroscopes, all relatively new at the time.

At that time, Crawford Long did not have a GI laboratory, so Rubye David and the operating room staff gave him a place to work—a treatment room in the OR. He had one nurse to assist him. The small, crowded space became "a total nuisance to the operating room," so the way was made to make a GI laboratory under the "impetus of Robert Tharpe, Pollard Turman, Frank Swift, Henry Bowden, Charles West, and Boisfeuillet Jones."

Dr. Davis said, "When my Daddy died, these men decided they wanted to name something in his honor. They knew how proud he was that we were able to provide this type of diagnostic service at Crawford Long Hospital and they were really the impetus behind raising the seed money."

Dr. Davis said, "These business people from Atlanta went out and bought all the [needed] instruments; the business community made the monetary commitment to start the GI laboratory at Crawford Long. I was very impressed with how these very busy people would spend their time and show interest in a local hospital with their recurring gifts." Members of Dr. Davis' family also contributed to the fund.

Today, gifts are earmarked for educational purposes. The hospital now takes care of all capital expenditures, the buying and servicing of equipment.

Dr. Davis remembers when only an occasional patient was treated. Now patients from all over the country, and especially in the Southeast, are referred to Crawford Long for specialized procedures. "With the use of laser and papillatomes, special electrical probes and dilating devices, we could stop bleeding, seal blood vessels, open narrow places, close broken places. All this could be accomplished through our instruments. A boon! Particularly for an older patient who might not do well with a general anesthetic or open abdominal surgery.

"Whoever heard, in the early 1970s, of a person having a gallbladder attack with a gallstone in the bile duct swallowing a thing with a light beam on it, having a little opening made and a balloon put in to pull out a gallstone, and then let the patient go home in the afternoon? Yet it's routine now." How different from the gallstone operation performed by Dr. Fischer on the opening day of the Davis-Fischer Sanatorium in 1911.

Dr. Davis points with pride to the use of a laser beam to seal up a bleeding ulcer, allowing the patient to go home in about two days. The same operation in the 1970s meant a minimum two-week stay in the hospital for treatment. "I think of the impact of just what we at Crawford Long have seen in the cost effectiveness of this particular procedure in how fast it gets people out of the hospital and how much money it saves for everyone. Fiberoptic endoscopy has totally revolutionized the field.

"Somewhere between 1972-73, with this endoscope, we were able to remove a quarter from a young child without surgery," recalls Dr. Davis. "I remember Dr. Murdock Equen had his magnet back in the '40s had removed a coin from the body of a child. Now there isn't enough metal in our coins for the magnet to pick them up. So we devised a way to remove this foreign body from the child. We made a special wire to go around the quarter to remove it. I didn't think much about it then, but Rubye David told me this was the first time such a thing had been done," said Dr. Davis.

It received national attention, including mention on the "Paul Harvey" and "Today" shows. Major newspapers picked up the story from the wire services.

In 1986, an AIDS victim bleeding from a colon tumor was treated with laser to rid him of the cancer. This was a new development of the early treatment of cancer with laser.

Another of Dr. Davis' interesting cases deals with a football-size blockage in the stomach of a patient. Dr. J.D. Martin, observing the operation to remove it, noted: "That is a gastric phytobezoar. I don't think I have ever seen but one or two in my entire career." Dr. Davis was amused when his next patient had exactly the same problem, prompting Dr. Martin to say, "You have increased my experience 100% in a couple of hours."

Later, while observing the use of tenderizer on a steak in a backyard cookout, Dr. Davis had the idea that the same tenderizing action might be duplicated on a bezoar. From subsequent research, he learned there was agreement that a "bezoar would have to be cut out." He decided he would try the tenderizer. It proved successful with seven patients, so he wrote and published an article on it for the Journal of the American Medical Association.

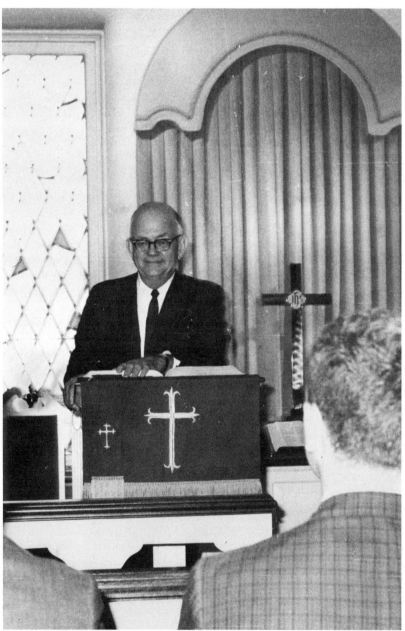

Reverend Huckaby in the hospital chapel.

CHAPEL PROGRAM

Mr. Shelley Davis spoke at the Fiftieth Anniversary of the Crawford Long Hospital Nursing School on June 6, 1958, and closed out his tribute to the nurses with the following words:

"My father [Dr. E. C. Davis] would have been proud to see the present institution in which he had such a part in its early life. Both he and Dr. Fischer, were they alive, would be busy planning for an even greater future to fit the times. Perhaps the future may even hold chaplain service at Crawford Long as is the practice in other Atlanta hospitals to meet the needs of our times."

This was an idea whose time had come. Doctors understand the need for a place apart where family members of seriously ill patients or staff members with personal problems can retreat for respite. They are aware of the tensions present in waiting rooms where anxious relatives sit for hours, pondering hopeful or despairing information until they feel hemmed in by anxiety, weariness and apprehension.

A chapel can provide an oasis in the busy hospital routine. It's a place to go for prayer, for renewed strength to meet whatever the next hours will bring.

Crawford Long now has such a chapel—a set-aside place whose soft decor lends itself to rest and contemplation—on the ground floor of the Davis-Fischer building, just off the lobby.

Soon after a place for the Chapel was set aside, the Crawford Long Auxiliary raised $10,000 to provide furnishing of the newest addition to the hospital complex. This amount represented 5,500 hours of volunteer work, some from the profits of the Auxiliary gift shop and from the hospitality cart earnings.

Bishop John Owen Smith officiated at the Chapel dedication

ceremonies on October 22, 1961. He was assisted by Dr. W. Rembert Sisson.

Light filters in through windows of small diamond-shaped panes glazed in pastel colors, falls from a skylight that lets sunshine in like a spirit of hope. Pews and kneelers, cushioned in rose-colored velvet, match the curved draping of the altar backdrop and altar cloth. Two lighted candles flank an open Bible.

Nurses, doctors and friends of Caroline Estelle Ward contributed to a special memorial fund for the altar cloths and other furnishings to honor her memory. Miss Ward, who joined the Crawford Long staff as a nursing supervisor in 1944, resigned in 1960. A "lifetime nurse," she was a graduate of the Class of 1925.

To one side of the altar is an organ given in memory of Mildred Baggett, RN, Class of 1926, by her family. Pine-flecked marble floors and side trim add dignity and strength to the atmosphere; earth brown carpeting softens footfalls. A table at the rear, just under a picture of John Wesley holding the hand of a child as he looks with compassion at a crippled man and the child's mother, holds copies of "Upper Room" and "Guideposts."

A plaque dated 1961 tells of gratitude and appreciation to the Auxiliary of Crawford Long Hospital for its generosity in equipping the Chapel. Another, dated 1971, says: "Chapel refurbished by the family and friends in memory of Hyman B. Stillerman, M.D., through the generosity of the Auxiliary of the Crawford Long Hospital."

Red hymnals and copies of blue New Testaments with Psalms, placed by the Gideons, provide material in the pews for meditation.

The Chapel ministry began in the spring of 1960 when the medical staff made a formal request to Dr. Glenn to provide chaplain service to Crawford Long. They asked for an experienced pastor to fill the position. Bishop Moore, head of the North Georgia Conference of the United Methodist Church, appointed the Rev. Louis F. Huckaby to the office of the new chaplain program.

Chaplain Huckaby began his work July 1, 1960, in an empty office. So he started walking down the halls, stopping to call on patients. He continued this practice of daily calls as long as he worked at Crawford Long. In what he described as the "most enriching experience that ever came into my thirty years of ministry," he saw the program expand.

A secretary, Gaynelle Newton, herself the wife of a minister, was employed. When Mrs. Newton's husband assumed a pastorate in Alabama, a new secretary was hired. After three temporary helpers came and went, Mrs. Sara Hyde, who worked elsewhere in the hospital for twelve years, came to work in the office.

For many years thereafter, Mrs. Hyde served not only as Chaplain Huckaby's secretary and office assistant, but also as the Chapel organist. Her daily recitals were eagerly anticipated by staff and patients, and inspired this poem by Nancy Yarn:

The Hospital Chapel Organ

When the world is too much with you
And you weary of its ways
Just stop a moment and listen
As the Chapel organ plays-
The strains of soft, sweet music
Will soothe each jangled nerve
And you'll put the words to each clear note
"How Blessed are Those Who Serve"
Your voice will lose its strident tones
And a smile will start to form
As you hum the music, sing the words
"Lord, Take my Hand and Lead Me Home"
And as you listen you grow serene
And peace returns to you-
And you wish, as the chords sound sweetly there
That everyone could listen, too

Mrs. Hyde, whose music was such delight to patients and staff members for twelve years, is still making music. Now a resident of Lakewood Manor in the Sylvan Hills community, she plays the piano for Sunday School and Wednesday night prayer meetings. She also plays for the Lakewood Manor choir where she celebrated her 79th birthday in September 1986.

Over the years, special services have filled the chapel pews. When President John F. Kennedy was assassinated, a service was held in his memory. Chaplain Huckaby recalls he presided at four funeral services in memory of Dr. Martin Luther King, Jr. so all employees would be able to pay their respects. On the day of Dr. King's death, administration received a number of early morning calls asking that all employees be relieved of their duties to attend the King funeral. Because it wasn't possible to have so many employees from all departments away from duty, it was decided that every employee would be allowed to attend an appropriate service.

Weddings, too, became a part of the program as many student nurses, far away from home, were married in the Chapel during their school days. Employees, too, have chosen the Crawford Long Chapel as the setting for their nuptials.

Of his years of work at Crawford Long, Chaplain Huckaby said, "Over half of my life and ministry have been spent in Atlanta and I've met a lot of people. At least a half million people went through this hospital as patients during the years I was here. A great big chunk of my heart's love is at Crawford Long."

The Rev. Fred L. Glisson, a retired minister who had served four Atlanta Methodist churches plus nine years as a chaplain at Emory Hospital came to Crawford Long as an assistant chaplain on July 1, 1968.

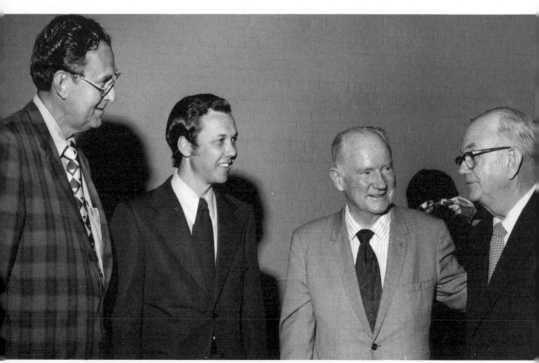

Chaplain Huckaby (far right) discusses retirement plans with Mr. Daniel Barker, Chaplain Jim Winn and Dr. Glenn.

When Chaplain Huckaby retired in June of 1972, his successor was the Rev. Jim Winn.

"Jim is like a son to me," Chaplain Huckaby said. Chaplain Winn, described as "a young man who cares about people and enjoys ministering them" was excited to assume his new duties July 1, 1972, just when the hospital was opening the new building. Chaplain Winn stayed at Crawford Long for ten years, and was followed by the Rev. Frank Jenkins who served two years.

The Rev. Harold D. Jones came to Crawford Long in June 1984. "At that time," he said, "Mr. Henry asked me to be a pastor to the staff as well as to the patients and their families. This is the direction my ministry is focused, on the staff."

Chaplain Jones said that in addition to the Chapel there is a Quiet Room on each floor of the hospital, where families can discuss matters with physicians or chaplains. He smiled as he added, "Sometimes we, or the doctors, step into a Quiet Room for a moment to gather our own thoughts."

There is also spacious room on the third floor of the hospital, where a family can wait while a loved one is in surgery. The family waiting room was established by the Crawford Long Auxiliary in 1981 when Mrs. Vonetta Ramos was the chairperson. This project had the wholehearted support of Dr. Glenn, who helped coordinate the colors and furniture for the room.

Nina Fleeman, an Auxiliary volunteer, explained that the comfortable room is there to help while away the hours of waiting. Plants, a rack of recent magazines and puzzles, plus a small kitchen that provides tea, coffee or hot chocolate gives a homey touch to those awaiting word of a family member's progress. Telephones are there to accept incoming or outgoing calls. Mrs. Fleeman said the chaplains often stop by to talk with those waiting, to offer them words ofen couragement or to just listen.

On January 1, 1986, the Reverend Elwood H. Spackman was appointed Director of Chaplaincy Services at Crawford Long Hospital and Associate Director of Pastoral Services for Emory University Affiliated Hospitals by Bishop Ernest Fitzgerald.

Chaplain Spackman brought the experience of nineteen years in the pastorate of North Georgia and South Carolina, a Master of Divinity degree from the Candler School of Theology at Emory, and advanced clinical pastoral training. On May 15, 1987, Chaplain Spackman was moved into the position of Administrator for Emory University Affiliated Hospitals.

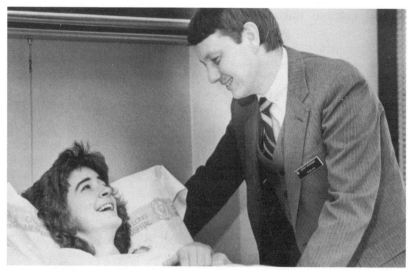

Chaplain Woody Spackman visits his daughter Julie in the Outpatient Center.

Chaplain Harold Jones was promoted to Director of Pastoral Services at Crawford Long and Associate Director of Pastoral Services, Emory University Affiliated Hospitals, and Chaplain Emily Sessions became Associate Director and Coordinator of Staff Support Services.

The Rev. Emily Sessions joined Crawford Long in November 1986. She is a graduate of Florida State University and Candler School of Theology at Emory University. She completed her clinical pastoral education at Grady Hospital in 1979. Prior to her coming to Crawford Long, she served as chaplain and director of pastoral care for seven years at Hamilton Medical Center in Dalton, Georgia.

Her ministry's goal is to help colleagues discover or develop their own resources for sustaining each other and themselves through times of high-stress in the task of health care. Rev. Jones said, "We do this through individual work with people, counseling and helping with referrals; we do this through working in staff-support groups. These groups provide a place for people to meet with each other in the midst of their working together and reclaim the value of the community they share. The result of these discoveries is a kind of power and healing that comes from caring for others and knowing others care for you."

Working in the clinical program with the staff chaplains are ten full-time students from the Candler School of Theology. The students work six hours a week at the hospital, visiting patients and meeting with supervisors as part of their pastoral training. Other assistants, working on programs similar to graduate study, work forty hours a week for credit and further experience that will enlarge their outreach.

Chaplain Jones said, "There is always a chaplain on call twenty-four hours a day. For convenience and easy availability at night, an apartment is maintained for the chaplain on night duty. A beeper is provided. Should a crisis arise, a nurse immediately alerts the chaplain."

Regular worship services are conducted in the Chapel every Sunday; Christmas, Easter and special days are marked with appropriate services. Once a year, a memorial service is conducted in honor of staff members who died in the preceding twelve months.

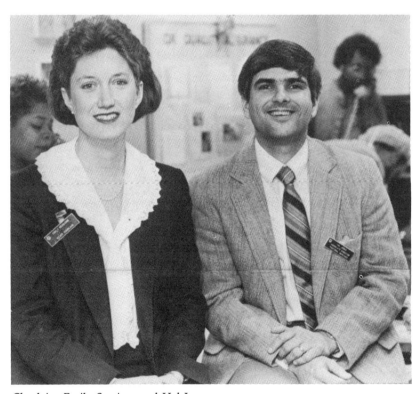

Chaplains Emily Sessions and Hal Jones.

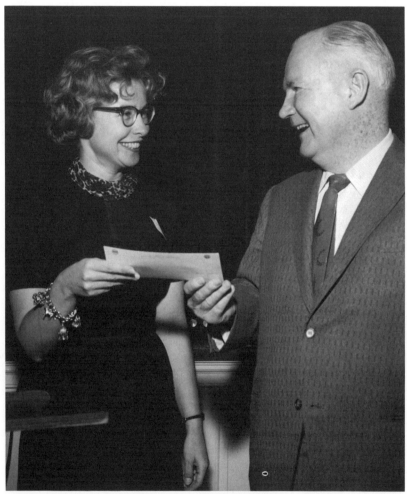

Mrs. J. H. Elrod, Jr., President of the Auxiliary, presents a check for $30,000 to Dr. Glenn. The money was raised in 1964 as part of a three-year pledge by the Auxiliary.

THE AUXILIARY
TO THE CRAWFORD LONG
HOSPITAL

Volunteers served as nurses' aides during World War II under the banner of the Red Cross. Pictures in the scrapbooks housed in the hospital museum show Mrs. Robert Woodruff at work in an operation observation post. Another pictures Mrs. William A. Hardmon and Mrs. Frank M. Curry pushing a baby "train" made up of seven cribs holding seven infants bound for their mothers' arms. Another shows Virginia Dulaney and Louise McCauley reading to small patients in the Pediatric Department.

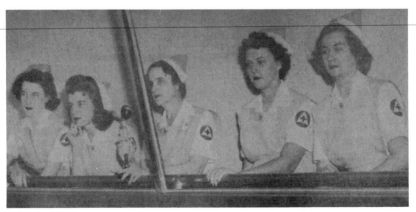

Behind glass in the operating room observation post, Nurses'
Aides Virginia Dulaney, LaRue Mizell, Mrs. Robert Woodruff,
Mrs. George R. McCauley and Mrs. Richard Titus, left to right,
watch an operation. (Photo from the Atlanta Journal February 21, 1943).

Dr. Fischer expressed his gratitude for the work performed by the wartime volunteers when he said, "Expansion increased the need for nurses and volunteers. We owe a debt of gratitude to Civilian Defense and Red Cross workers who helped keep the hospital adequately staffed."

However, when the war ended, that volunteer program phased out.

In 1954, Margaret Clements had an idea to form a Woman's Auxiliary to serve Crawford Long Hospital with volunteer workers. Mrs. Clements, according to a record made by Mrs. James Brawner, gathered a group of ladies together to discuss the possibility of an auxiliary for Crawford Long. The organizational meeting, held on July 12, 1954, in the Nurses' Auditorium brought results. Mrs. Clement was elected temporary chairman and Mrs. Arthur Smith became secretary protem.

Among the 32 women present were Macie Stephens, Director of Nursing, and Georgia Belle Hearn Martin, Director of the Nursing Service. They explained a need for an auxiliary and offered their cooperation in starting one.

Charter members and officers were Mrs. George Williams; Mrs. William R. Crowe, Jr.; Mrs. Hugh G. Mosley; Mrs. J. C. Tanner; Mrs. J. L. Kurtz; Mrs. R. L. Robinson; Mrs. J. S. Reynolds; Mrs. A. A. Weinstein; Mrs. Worth Hobby; Mrs. Clifton Kemper; Mrs. Kells Boland; Mrs. D. T. Nabors; Mrs. James Weinberg; Mrs. Linton Bishop; Mrs. Frank Miles; Mrs. J. R. Simpson; Mrs. I. T. Shapiro; Mrs. A. A. Smith; Mrs. J. L. Clements, Jr.; Mrs. E. A. Allen; Mrs. J. W. Thompson; Mrs. E. M. Dunstan; Mrs. W. W. Daniel; Mrs. Richard Elmer; Mrs. J. W. Brawner, Sr.; Mrs. E. A. Bancker; Mrs. Shelley C. Davis; Mrs. Grattan Woodson; Mrs. Ben Read; Mrs. R. E. Boger; Mrs. J. R. Rogers; and Mrs. C. Richard King.

The Auxiliary's first list of regular officers consisted of Mrs. J. Luther Clements, president; Mrs. Richard Elmer, first vice-president; Mrs. Harry Wiley, second vice-president; Mrs. James I. Weinberg, recording secretary; Mrs. William R. Crowe, corresponding secretary; Mrs. Clifton Kemper, treasurer; and Mrs. Murray A. Howard, parliamentarian.

Membership was established in the American Hospital Association and bylaws were adopted stating the purpose of the organization—to provide service to the patients and to all members of the hospital staff. Bright pink uniforms and insignia identified the Auxiliary members as they moved into action.

Longtime members recall that the first "office" and the gift shop were squeezed into a tiny, windowless cubbyhole. A card table was the desk and a cigar box became a cash box. An old newspaper rack was used for displays. The gift shop stock was meager—a few boxes of candy, some chewing gum and a small supply of cigarettes.

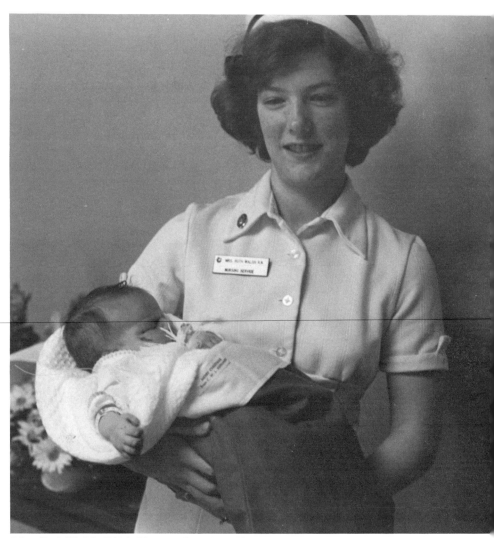

Mrs. Ruth Walsh, RN holds a newborn in a Christmas stocking provided by the Auxiliary.

This soon changed. Abrams Contractors donated the shop's first display case. Other gifts followed. The Newton Company gave candies, Lovable Brassiere Company contributed nursing bras and the Felton Supply Company presented toilet water, bath powder, and perfume sticks. Colonel Thompson of Thompson, Boland and Lee donated two display cases. Luke Swenson, associated with Sears, added valuable contributions. His company saw that a wall was removed to enlarge the working space and windows were installed on the corridor side. Two display cases, new shelves, and magazine racks added attractiveness and efficiency to the shop.

Crawford Long's Maintenance Department built a "Good Will Cart" to transport magazines, crackers, candy, and sundries directly to patients at their beds. Twice a week, volunteers bring cheery greetings and items for sale to patients. Today's "Cheer Cart" also holds flowers and balloons.

By the end of the second year, the gift shop offered toys, books, magazines, toilet articles, candies, crackers, and an ever-changing stock of get-well gifts and cards.

The revenue from these sales was used for purchases for the hospital and patients. The first year Auxiliary Christmas gift to the hospital was a television set and Christmas stockings filled with fruit and toys for the children in the Pediatric Department. To the delight of new mothers, their infants were tucked into large Christmas stockings for the babies' first trips out into the world.

Revenue from the gift shop, the Good Will Cart, bazaars, cake sales, and other projects funded the hospital chapel.

Auxiliary members, in addition to working with patients, became entrepreneurs, purchasing agents, decorators, bookkeepers and the compilers of a cookbook.

In the early 1970s, Mrs. Robert "Coc" Henson, Auxiliary chairman, and Mrs. Nancy Yarn became co-chairmen in the preparation of a cookbook, *Cooking With Love*. A box decorated by Cecil Lawton Easterly was placed in the cafeteria to receive favorite recipes from all hospital staff members as well as from Auxiliary members. Mr. Easterly also illustrated the cookbook cover. The McDaniel Printing Company printed *Cooking With Love* at a special rate. Mrs. Mona Temples and Miss Carolyn Bradley, staff members, acted as advisor and typist for the project.

In spite of hours of work by everyone, three errors crept into the final printout. Undaunted, the women saw to it the three recipes were retyped, cut down to page size, and pasted over the incorrect recipes. Mrs. Temples and her committee reworked the 5,000 copies of the cookbooks.

Members of the cookbook committee were Miss Dorothy Crawford, Miss Betty Dailey, Mrs. Laverne Elma, Mrs. C. Steadman Glisson, Mrs. James F. Olley, Mrs. Harold Ramos, and Mrs. James E. Short.

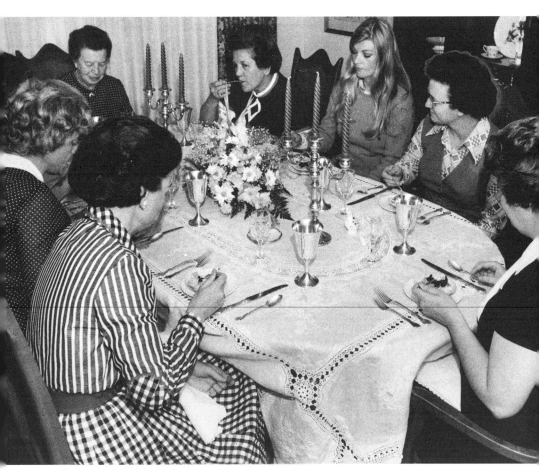

(Left to right) Mrs. J. F. Olley, Mrs. Laverne Elmer, Betty Dailey, Mrs. Nancy Yarn, Mrs. Mary Rollison, Mrs. J. F. Easterly Jr., Mrs. Mona Temples, and Mrs. Sybil Short sample recipes for the Crawford Long cookbook. (Photo from the Atlanta Journal/Constitution)

When male volunteers were added to the Auxiliary membership, the name was changed to "The Auxiliary to the Crawford Long Memorial Hospital," with Otis Barfield as its first male member. Marvin Bush, Cecil Downing, George Castleberry, Kay Kortkamp, John Matthews, and Harry Stein later joined the Volunteer roster.

In 1969, when plans to build the Peachtree Tower addition were announced, the Auxiliary pledged to give $100,000 to be paid out within a five-year period. This pledge was paid out within four years!

To raise such a large sum of money, the First Annual Crawford Long Ball was inaugurated, under the title "New Horizons." The annual dinner-dance has become a social tradition, raising funds for Auxiliary projects second only to gift shop revenue. This money has made possible renovations where needed, a fetal monitoring system, a breast imaging cancer center, a new surgical suite, contributions to the building fund, and the establishment of family rooms. Today a bright, large, and well-stocked gift shop is located in the Peachtree Tower.

As important as the monetary contribution is the personal service given by Auxiliary volunteers. Volunteers sort and deliver mail to patients, sometimes reading the messages on get-well cards or writing a letter for someone too ill to write. Others give TLC to children, rocking them in chairs donated to the Pediatrics Department by the Auxiliary. The School of Nursing is well acquainted with the Auxiliary. The Auxiliary has furnished music and refreshments for student dances and graduation receptions.

On Nurse's Day, the gift of pink carnations to the nurses adds sparkle to an otherwise routine day; a red carnation pinned to the jackets of hospital physicians on Doctor's Day brings smiles. Auxiliary hostesses serve refreshments at retirement parties and they are present for memorial services.

The Auxiliary members take pride that one of their number was selected for recognition by the American Hospital Association in 1986. Mrs. Robert "Coc" Henson, an active member for over twenty-five years and twice president during that time, was presented a certificate recognizing her service.

Later that year, a letter from WXIA-TV 11 chose her to receive the Community Service Award, a Jefferson Award for public service, and $1,000 to be given to the charity of her choice. The award, presented April 22, 1986, was the first such honor paid to a member of the Crawford Long Auxiliary. Mrs. Henson chose to present the $1,000 to the Physical Therapy Department.

When she received the awards from WXIA-TV, Mrs. Henson said, "These awards are for all the Auxiliary members. Everyone has worked hard to bring about the accomplishments for which they are given."

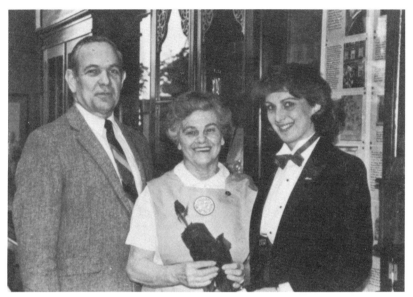

Caption: Mrs. Robert "Coc" Henson pictured here with Mr. Henry and Robin Conklin of WXIA-TV, Channel 11, was chosen to receive one of ten 1986 11-Alive Community Service Awards

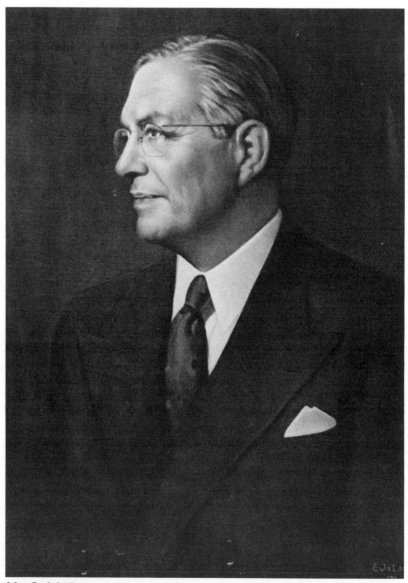

Mr. Carlyle Fraser

CARLYLE FRASER HEART CENTER

The Carlyle Fraser Heart Center of Crawford Long Hospital was established for the prevention, care, treatment, and correction of heart disease, the number one killer in the United States.

The Center, divided into cardiology, pulmonary medicine, and thoracic and cardiovascular sections, contains the most sophisticated equipment for diagnosis and treatment available. This includes cardiac catheterization, myocardial nuclear scanning, echocardiology and phonocardiography equipment.

The Carlyle Fraser Heart Center was established through the philanthropy of the family and friends of the late Carlyle Fraser, founder and executive of Genuine Auto Parts.

The dedication of the Carlyle Fraser Heart Center, established in his memory, took place February 22, 1976 in the auditorium of the Agnes Raoul Glenn Memorial Building. Bishop William R. Cannon opened the Act of Dedication. Dr. Sanford Atwood, President of Emory University, presided and the Rev. Dr. Harry Fifield pronounced the invocation. Dr. Linton H. Bishop, Jr., member of the Emory Board of Trustees and a member of the Crawford Long staff, welcomed guests.

After a showing of the film, "The Carlyle Fraser Heart Center," Dr. Glenn accepted the Center as a part of the Crawford Long complex and Bishop Cannon offered the dedication litany. Responses to this were made by the Honorable George Busbee, Governor of Georgia and the Honorable Thomas B. Murphy, Speaker of the Georgia House of Representatives. The Rev. Jim Winn, Crawford Long chaplain, pronounced the benediction to the service attended by Mrs. Carlyle Fraser, widow of Mr. Fraser, and members of her family.

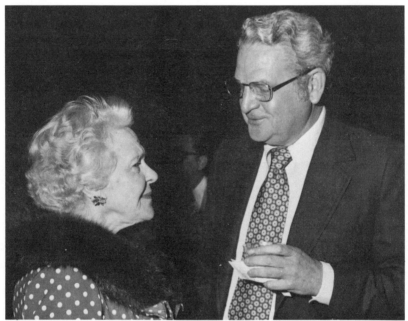

Mrs. Carlyle Fraser and Mr. William C. Hatcher,
President of Genuine Parts Company.

Two floors of the Crawford Long Peachtree Building are set aside for patients utilizing the facilities of cardiac catheterization, echocardiography, myocardial nuclear scanning, and phonocardiography.

A surgical suite for all types of heart and blood vessel surgery including open heart operations and patient care area with two intensive care areas for acute coronary care patients are also a part of the Center. In March of 1979, the Fraser Center became the first medical facility in Atlanta to acquire a mobile scintillation camera and computer.

"The saving of lives is tremendous," said Dr. R. Bruce Logue, the Heart Center's Director. Dr. Logue's national reputation as a teacher and cardiologist has led to the establishment of the Bruce Logue Chair of Cardiology by the Emory Board of Trustees in March 1986. He was a founding member and the first president of the Georgia Heart Association. Dr. Logue holds weekly conferences on diagnosis and treatment of heart disease and related dysfunctions and lung disorders.

The Center's work continues through the generosity and ongoing support of the family and friends of Carlyle Fraser. Mr. Wilton Looney, Chairman of the Board of Genuine Parts Company, like the late Mr. Fraser, has an abiding interest in philanthropy and a special friendship with the Carlyle Fraser Center.

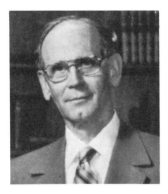

Wilton Looney, chairman of Genuine Parts Co., has provided leadership that has shaped The Carlyle Fraser Heart Center.

Under the leadership of Dr. Linton H. Bishop, Jr., Dr. Charles R. Hatcher, Jr., and Mr. Looney, the Fraser Center continues to grow and play an important role in medical affairs in the Southeast. The Center trains medical personnel in clinical cardiology through the Emory University School of Medicine Affiliated Hospital Training Program.

Over a six-month period in 1984, over 2,000 open heart procedures were performed without a single fatality. This included coronary bypass, valve replacement, and other operations. To celebrate this achievement, members of the cardiac team were given a reception and an opportunity to hear Dr. Alain Carpenter, noted French cardiovascular surgeon. Over 100 people were present.

Another heart-healing story began as a result of observations by Dr. Andreas Gruentzig and led to the discovery of the coronary angioplastic "balloon" procedure. Dr. Gruentzig, originally from Switzerland and associated with Emory University Hospital and Crawford Long, devised the "balloon catheter" as the result of a casual remark by a patient suffering a coronary obstruction. "Do you have to open the chest?" the patient inquired. "Why don't you just ream it out?"

"That gave me an idea," said Dr. Gruentzig later. During research, he learned of a technique discovered by Dr. Charles Dotter. Dr. Dotter, while performing an angiogram on a patient, penetrated a stenosis area with a catheter which opened a new channel the size of the catheter where the artery had been blocked. Dr. Gruentzig observed this procedure in Germany, thought about it, began work on refining it in Switzerland using laboratory animals.

In 1971, he used it on the leg of a human being. By 1973, he had refined it for pelvic arteries. He continued to perfect the process until 1977, when he introduced the balloon catheter on the heart of a patient.

Since then, thousands of patients have benefitted from Dr. Gruentzig's treatment for arteries narrowed by plaque deposits. When the tiny balloon is inflated, it pushes the plaque back, freeing blood flow. Doctors call it "percutaneous transluminal coronary angioplasty." About 10 to 15 percent of coronary patients are candidates for this angioplastic procedure.

The Cardiac Catheterization Laboratory (Cath Lab) of the Fraser Center received an award in recognition of 1,000 angioplasties performed over a 5-year period. The Cath Lab completed its 1,000th angioplasty on August 12, 1985. Currently, approximately 30 to 40 such procedures are done every month.

Another facet of Fraser people at work is the publishing of 50 articles or book chapters in national medical journals and publications including the textbook *The Heart*. Authors of these published papers are Dr. Robert Guyton, Dr. Willis Williams, Dr. Gilbert Grossman, Dr. Joseph Miller, Dr. Gerald Staton, Dr. Douglas Morris, Dr. Henry Liberman, Dr. Louis Batty, Dr. Randolph Patterson, Dr. Andre Churchwell, and Lynne Dorsey, RN. Several papers and abstracts have been presented at national meetings.

Another ongoing project supported by the Carlyle Fraser Heart Center is the work of the Pulmonary Function Laboratory headed by Dr. Gilbert Grossman. The pulmonary section of the Fraser Center is recognized for its high quality respiratory care, its diagnosis, treatment, and management of respiratory diseases. Patients from other hospitals receive treatment via a computer linkup to the Pulmonary Lab. Referrals are made to it throughout the South.

Physician Assistants (PAs) play a vital role at the Fraser Center. They have completed the highest level of training in their field and carry the board-certified identification of PAC (Physician Assistant Certified).

Back in its beginning, the Fraser Center performed approximately 40 catheterizations a month. By 1986, that average had jumped to more than 100. The number of open heart operations rose leaped

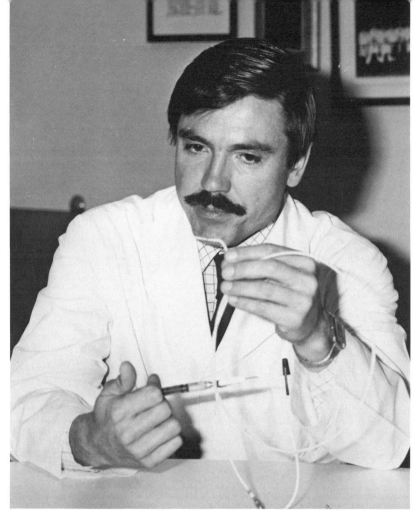

Dr. Andreas Gruentzig

to 450 in 1985, in contrast to 50 performed the first year.

Costs for Fraser Center patients who voluntarily participate in research diagnostic procedures are supported by grants from various organizations and from special funds.

In the spring of the 10th Anniversary year of the existence of the Carlyle Fraser Heart Center, Mr. John D. Henry said, "The Center is recognized as one of the premier cardiac centers in the country. The importance of the Carlyle Fraser Heart Center will grow steadily as we continue to conduct groundbreaking research and develop new procedures and improve existing ones."

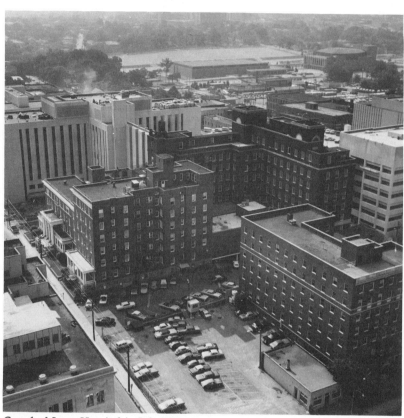

Crawford Long Hospital in July 1973

C H A P T E R   T W E L V E

FURTHER
EXPANSION

Crawford Long Hospital, by the end of 1986, was the second largest hospital in Atlanta. Growth at Crawford Long has been maintained through crises, building construction, and temporary setbacks. Issues have been met as they arose, problems were confronted and solved.

In the spring of 1967, Atlanta faced hospital bed shortages, a lack of registered and practical nurses, laboratory technologists, dietitians, physical therapists, and occupational therapists. This shortage of health care workers caused an upsurge in wages and posed a problem for all hospital business departments.

Mr. Daniel Barker observed that increased wage demands hit hospitals twice as hard as similar demands to industry, where payroll monies comprise about a third of overall operation costs. "For example," he said, "the impact of a $10 wage increase for hospital personnel would result in a seven dollar increase in a patient's bill." The rise in nurses' salaries is one example of rising costs. In 1965, the starting salary for a nurse was $325 a month. By 1967, it had increased to $450-475 a month.

Also cited among escalating hospital costs was the increase of laundry, recordkeeping, housekeeping, maintenance, dietary and pharmacy rates, and the costs of new equipment.

HOME HEALTH CARE PLAN INITIATED

By July of 1968, it was apparent that the hospital stays could be shortened and costs cut if ways could be found to provide follow-up home care. A community effort brought forth a pilot study called "Trial 33." Held at St. Joseph's Infirmary, it was sponsored by the Community Council of the Atlanta Area, Inc.

The thrust of the plan was to direct the patient to the proper kind of care at the right time, using all available facilities, personnel and services. The study sought answers: Will doctors refer patients? Can existing facilities, such as the Visiting Nursing Association and public health services, provide needed home care?

Results of the "Trial 33" study proved answers to these questions were, for the most part, affirmative. It was calculated that the study at St. Joseph's Infirmary saved ninety-two days of hospital care for about eleven of thirty-three patients in the project.

Agencies involved with "Trial 33" were V.A., Public Health, Easter Seal Society, Home Rehabilitation, Cancer Society, sixteen institutions and twenty-seven doctors.

Crawford Long became one of two hospitals that initiated the home health care plan with hospital coordinators employed on full- or part-time basis. Linda Durham, RN, serving as Crawford Long coordinator, saw and referred patients to public health, rehabilitation and child welfare agencies. She told of giving applicable advice to a diabetic. She said, "We tell the patient and the family about the importance of diet control. We notify the Diabetic Association; we teach the patient about injections he/she will have to use upon discharge." She emphasized proper teaching in the beginning would save hospital bed use and cut down on repeated hospitalization. Financing for the care would be absorbed by agencies such as the United Way or Medicare.

LAUNDRY EXPANSION

The Laundry Department, rated "excellent" month after month by the American Institute of Laundries, could look with pride at new machinery in 1974.

Steve Paugh showed the installation of three new washing machines, each with a capacity load of 600. A new automatic sheet folder, capable of folding sixty sheets a minute, added efficiency to maintaining a four-change supply of linen at all times: fresh linen on the floor, two fresh stacks in the linen room, and one in the laundry.

GIFT FOR LIFE

On May 17, 1971, the Gift For Life program was launched to

raise funds for needed expansion at costs an estimated at $28 million. Financing for the program was to come partly from gifts by friends. A $10 million loan commitment was made to add to an "on hands" fund amounting to $2 million. The steering group was headed by Pollard Turman. Other committee members were Henry Bowden, William R. Bowdoin, James Sibley, Rankin Smith, and Dr. Robert W. Candler.

The program included a $16 million nine floor patient addition, a radiation therapy center, and the modernization of patient care facilities in existing hospital buildings.

The Gift For Life drive had, as its stated aim, the continued ability to give individual care to patients, and to maintain the goals of Dr. Davis and Dr. Fischer when they founded the hospital—to provide the most advanced therapy available at the least cost to the patient.

By January 17, 1972, Dr. Linton H. Bishop, Jr., General Chairman of the Gift For Life program, was able to announce the initial goal of $4 million in gifts had been met.

NEW RADIATION DEPARTMENT

Among the goals was establishment of the Radiation Center on Prescott Street to provide cancer treatment in a time when there was a critical shortage of such units. Ground was broken for the Agnes Raoul Glenn Memorial Building in December of 1971. This building, which houses the Radiation Therapy Department, was given by the Glenn Foundation as a memorial to the mother of Dr. Wadley Glenn and Mr. Wilbur Glenn.

Dr. Murray Copeland, noted cancer specialist and Assistant Director of the University of Texas M. D. Anderson Hospital and Tumor Institute, spoke at the ground breaking.

The new building would connect with the central hospital complex by a tunnel running under Prescott Street, and house the Department of Nuclear Medicine, a new library, conference and lecture rooms, plus five floors for offices for faculty, house staff, and private physicians.

The Radiation Center opened in November 1973. Dr. Glenn welcomed guests to the dedication on November 12. Chaplain Winn pronounced the invocation. Dr. J. D. Martin introduced the speaker, Dr. Claude E. Welsh, President of the American College of Surgeons. Mr. Dan Barker closed the ceremony of dedication.

The multi-million dollar center's equipment included a co-balt 65 Unit with a high output of approximately 15 million volts of energy of gamma rays. At the time, it provided the treatment used for most cancer patients. There were two other x-ray units, a conventional and a superficial unit.

EMERGENCY ROOM

In 1974, Dr. Harold S. Ramos, Director of Medical Education, cited a need for improvement in the outgrown Crawford Long Emergency Department. "There are only three places to see people," he said. "There are three beds and no waiting room facilities. People not critically ill have to wait on stretchers in the hall. There is no room for a lab or x-ray equipment, no storage place." Staff doctors added their dissatisfaction with the cramped quarters, lack of privacy, and general confusion when the number of patients multiplied.

"Emergency care has changed in the past twenty years," said Dr. Ramos. "Before, after hours you would call a doctor and meet him at his office or he could make house calls. Now doctors meet patients in the Emergency Department because that's where the equipment is located. You can no longer carry what you need in a little black bag."

Because of its central location, Crawford Long has a large potential emergency population. Weekdays, there is the central Atlanta working population, as well as conventioneers with emergency care needs to be met. Close-in city dwellers also look to Crawford Long for treatment. The Emergency Room also serves people without a regular doctor.

The Emergency staff is ready to meet their needs. Like all emergency departments, Crawford Long uses triage (assigning priorities of medical treatment on the basis of urgency or chance for survival). People in life or death situations are treated first. Those in less critical circumstances may have to wait for treatment. Weekends and early evening hours are the busiest times for the Emergency Room, which is open twenty-four hours a day.

A coronary observation radio enables communication between the Emergency Department and medics en route to the hospital.

These improvements were made possible in part by funds from the Crawford Long Auxiliary and the Mary Allen Lindsey Branan Foundation. In 1973, the emergency rooms were staffed by two full-time physicians. In 1976, space went from 800 to 3,300 square feet to include four examination rooms, one minor surgery room, a trauma room, a cardiac room and an orthopedic room. In a 1978 "Larynx" article, Dr. Cassandra Evans called the Emergency Room, "the window of the hospital."

The Emergency Department supports the annual Fourth of July Peachtree Road Race by standing ready in case runners need hospitalization. The hospital has developed its own t-shirt to give to those runners who come to the Emergency Room and do not finish the race. In 1985, Dr. Daniel Beless, Director of Emergency Medicine, gave out twenty-three tee shirts emblazoned with the hospital's name as consolation prizes to disappointed runners who were brought to Crawford Long in distress. Dr. Beless said, "Most of them were more concerned over not getting a race tee shirt than they were of their own physical condition. We hope the tee shirt we gave them eased some of their pain."

When people arrive at the emergency door, they are often in pain and are frightened. In May of 1986, an elderly woman struck down by a backing automobile was brought in bearing bruises and sustaining a broken arm. Her waiting time was short, and she left the hospital feeling she had been treated well. Her recovery was rapid and uneventful. Before that, she'd resented emergency room treatment she and her children had received elsewhere, but she said her resentment evaporated in view of the care she received at Crawford Long.

GYNECOLOGY AND OBSTETRIC GIFT

Anne Winship Bates Leach and her husband, Willaford Ransom Leach, honored Dr. Wadley Glenn, Dr. George Williams, and Dr. John McCain by presenting a gift of $1 million to Crawford Long Hospital in May 1975. The income from this trust was designated for improvement of the Gynecology and Obstetrics Departments and for cancer research.

The Leachs were elected first honorary members of the attending staff at Crawford Long in February 1976. This honor was presented by Dr. Cullen Richardson.

MARGARET BROWN HATCHER CENTER

The Margaret Brown Hatcher Nursing Education Center,

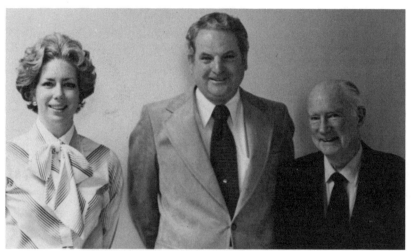

Dr. Wadley R. Glenn tours the Margaret Brown Hatcher Nursing Education Center with Mr. Hatcher and his daughter Peggy.

established in memory of Mrs. Margaret Brown Hatcher, was opened in March 1977. The Hatcher Center, located on the 6th floor of the Davis-Fischer Building, was made possible by the generosity of Mrs. Hatcher's husband, William Hatcher, and her family and friends. It was developed to provide an education area for patients and nursing service personnel separate from the clinical working areas.

This new center houses a teaching lab for training bedside skills for both patients and staff, a hundred seat classroom and a smaller classroom, a resource room and office space.

A new nursing service employee, after general and specialized orientation, here learns hospital policies, procedures and expectations, helping insure a more competent nurse and a more confident employee. This program was designed to keep nurses up-to-date on new and expanding nursing care programs and new techniques, equipment, facilities and concepts of care.

ENGINEERING DEPARTMENT

Keeping a hospital warm in winter and cool in summer, and making sure that water flows, lights burn, and machinery works is not a dramatic medical miracle, but in some cases, life itself depends on these uninterrupted services.

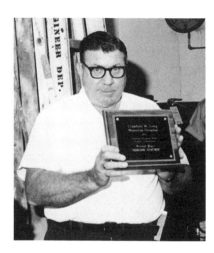

Mr. William Moore holds an award won by the Engineering Department in a 1979 National Hospital Week competition.

As the hospital plant expanded, the work of William Moore, Chief Engineer and Director, has been divided into specialized department areas: the main plant, general maintenance, electrical maintenance and biomedical equipment, television and electronics, construction, painting, plumbing and stock room.

A staff of five, under supervision of John Wilkie, oversees the main steam plant and boilers, which make steam for all sterilizing equipment, and provide hot water for labs and operating rooms. Two hundred and fifty electric motors drive pumps, fans and actuator motors.

A significant addition to the physical plant was the construction of a helipad, begun in the spring of 1985 and officially opened in December of 1985. It was built on the fifth level of the Prescott Street parking deck.

Looking down from the 8th floor of the Woodruff Building, one can get a bird's eye view of the seventy by seventy foot landing pad marked with a large squared cross. Centered in the cross is a large "H" outlined in a six inch red line to give greater visibility. A large figure 5 warns incoming pilots the pad holds up to a five-ton helicopter.

A door from the heliport leads into the fourth floor of the Glenn Building where elevators can transport patients directly to the Emergency Rooms. Patients have been landed on the helipad from other area hospitals and from as far away as Charlotte, North Carolina.

The general maintenance section keeps lights lit, wheels and doorknobs turning. Cliff Wyatt, Supervisor of the biomedical and electronics shop, oversees all electrical repairs. James Head makes certain all TV and in-house communications systems are functioning. Jesse Holmes has the responsibility of 1500 bathrooms including inside and outside sewer lines. He also sees to repairs of dietary and laundry equipment. Hundreds of items in the storeroom are dispensed by Nancy Zawrotney while Mary Lancaster handles incoming work requests, records and clerical needs.

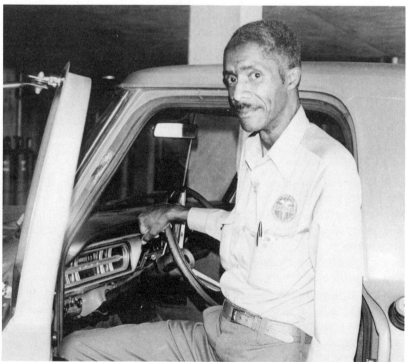

Long-time employee Mr. Warner Ward.

Mr. Moore had special words of praise for the late Warner Ward, a long-time employee of the department. "We used to say the place would shut down if it weren't for Warner," said Mr. Moore.

Maintenance costs have also risen, Mr. Moore said, "Ten years ago a doorknob cost thirty dollars, now it costs ninety to replace one."

REAL ESTATE GROWTH

In April 1986, 2.4 acres of land along West Peachtree were purchased. This former site of John Smith Chevrolet was bought to enlarge parking space for hospital employees. The former car showroom was set aside for renovation into The Carlyle Fraser Heart Center Research Laboratory.

In September 1986, property at 478-490 Peachtree Street was purchased. The building at 490 Peachtree has been renamed the Robert W. Candler Professional Building. The 478 Peachtree address will retain its original name, The W. W. Orr Doctors Building.

In December 1986, approximately two acres of land were sold to Citizens and Southern National Bank. Doctors Memorial Hospital on West Peachtree Street was bought the same day. With these acquisitions, Crawford Long gained 187 additional beds, parking space for 200 cars, 63,000 square feet of land and 162,000 square feet of hospital and office space.

CHANGING SPACES

In the same time period, the first phase of the Wadley Glenn Operating Pavilion was opened with four operating rooms, a new pharmacy and radiology facility.

The Woodruff Building has been extensively renovated, with three four-bed wards converted to semi-private rooms. This renovation of labor and delivery areas demonstrates Crawford Long Hospital's commitment to offer the most modern delivery techniques and care.

Future space reorganization includes moving the R. C. Davis GID Laboratory to more expansive quarters in the former Doctors Memorial Building.

During 1986, the number of residency positions increased from forty-five to fifty-two.

MORE PUBLIC OUTREACH

The Speakers Bureau was established as a community service program in November 1986. The Speakers Bureau offers speakers on health-related subjects at no cost to professional, civic, church, and service organizations in the Atlanta area.

For this program, more than fifty physicians and twenty-five staff members, including nurses, technicians, and therapists, will be available to speak on diabetes, cancer, obesity, nuclear cardiology, care for women, anemia, emotional issues related to cancer, AIDS, cardiology, health care service to the poor, African bush medicine, problems relating to alcoholics, health care in the U.S.S.R., death and dying, child psychiatry, surgery, impotence and physical therapy.

The Physician Referral Service, started in October 1986, is a free service to both the caller and the physician. It puts a patient who has no regular doctor in touch with a physician when a medical problem arises. This service is especially useful to new Atlantans, conventioneers, hotel visitors and people residing downtown.

Also in the line of service, Crawford Long developed some networking arrangements. During The Coca-Cola Company's Centennial Celebration, Crawford Long was its designated hospital. At the March meeting of the American College of Cardiology, the hospital provided on-site emergency medical service.

BIO-MEDICAL RESEARCH

Another development, involving the Carlyle Fraser Heart Center at Crawford Long and a new Bio-medical Technology Research Center established by Emory University and Georgia Institute of Technology, would have brought a smile to the face of Georgia Tech alumnus, Dr. Glenn.

Dr. Robert Guyton, Director of the Cardio-thoracic Research Laboratory of the Fraser Center and Associate Professor of Surgery at Emory, and Dr. Donald Giddens, Regent Professor of Mechanical Engineering at Georgia Tech, have been named directors of the new center.

In addition to providing an administrative structure for collaborational research and educational programing, Emory and Georgia Tech have committed $400,000 seed money a year through 1990.

FIRST STEPS

Crawford Long was chosen by groups of concerned persons to start a hospital-based program for new parents. The name "First

Steps" was given the project; it began officially in November 1984.

Crawford Long donated staff time and class space for six 2-1/2 hour training sessions for volunteers preparing to work with parents of healthy newborns. Dr. Anne Critz was chosen to teach an extended session to volunteers who would give longer term support to the parents of premature and other high-risk children.

Susan Bryant, First Steps Coordinator; Crawford Long Medical Social Worker, Sherry Buchanan; Chaplain Hal Jones, and Nurses Donna Galuki, Lydia McAllister, Judy McCook and Katherine Wright taught volunteers.

"First Steps" provided information and support to more than 15,000 families during its first thirteen months of activity. Sponsors were The Atlanta and DeKalb Junior Leagues, the Georgia Council of Child Abuse, the Atlanta Section of the National Council of Jewish Women and COPE (Coping with the Overall Pregnancy/Parenting Experience).

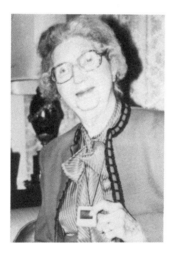

Ninety-three-year-old Mrs. Ruth Duckworth displays her Lifeline necklace.

LIFELINE

In an emergency, it is a necklace that can mean life or death to its elderly or shut-in wearer. It is called Lifeline.

In May 1986, the Lifeline program began at Crawford Long when the Atlanta Pilot Club members purchased materials for a response center in the Crawford Long Emergency Clinic, where trained workers are on duty twenty-four hours a day. There, signals are received from electronic boxes in patients' homes, alerting the hospital in an emergency.

Carolyn Anglin, Telecommunications Director, volunteers time to install the boxes she says gives their owners the "gift of independence." She said, "Lifeline allows [an elderly person] to live in . . . familiar surroundings with a secure feeling that help can be summoned in an instant at the pressing of a button. At the same time, the patient's caretaker is free of worry over a patient living alone."

Pressure on the necklace activates a unit under the patient's telephone. Alerted, a staff member immediately calls the subscriber whose name and address flashes on a receiving screen. Should this bring no response, a previously designated person is contacted to make a check on the caller.

Susana Jiminez, Community Relations Coordinator, directs this program. She interviews prospective Lifeline owners, installs units, and gives the simple instructions. The Crawford Long Auxiliary purchased several units for distribution, free of charge, to those who qualify. There is a monthly charge for the service.

OTHER OUTREACH PROGRAMS

Crawford Long, to help older adults in their efforts to keep healthy and active, joined the Adopt-A-High rise Program offering walking clubs and educational wellness projects to persons in selected retirement communities.

The walking clubs, the idea of the Atlanta Regional Commission's Pro Health For Seniors Task Force, are designed to combine fun and fitness. Crawford Long representatives meet with the seniors to give information on safe walking, what to wear and the correct effort needed.

As regional sponsor for the National Fitness Campaign's GAMEFIELDs, Crawford Long has helped in the construction of twenty GAMEFIELDs facilities at local schools, YMCAs, YWCAs and parks that applied for such facilities.

GAMEFIELDs provide jogging courses, trails with accompanying exercise sections, and fitness courses in limited areas designed to encourage body building, weight loss and cardiovascular conditioning. There are also walking courses for seniors and wheelchair sports courses for the physically handicapped.

A 10 Kilometer Run for Women was sponsored by Crawford Long in April 1987. A clinic to prepare the runners for the course was given by the Atlanta Track Club in January. In February, Crawford Long gave prospective runners a session on the nutrition needs for endurance. Five hundred women registered for the race. Despite the unseasonably cold and windy weather, 260 finished.

In November 1986, as part of a five-day cholesterol screening project sponsored by the American Health Foundation and WAGA-TV 5, Crawford Long joined other area hospitals to present community members with an opportunity to learn of their cholesterol levels. Each applicant was presented informative literature including a 'passport' in which to keep health records. The test was brief; results were reported after a short wait. Those with elevated cholesterol levels were advised to see their personal physicians.

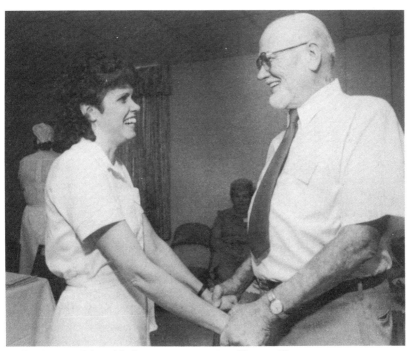

Cathy Rogers visits with former cancer patient Harvey Sharp at the first annual oncology reunion luncheon.

PATIENT REUNIONS

In September 1986, a second reunion of former Crawford

Long cancer patients in remission was held on the Woodruff Building veranda. Former patients, their families, nurses, doctors, administrators, chaplains and social workers "celebrated life and renewed health" together.

Ninety people were present, some from as far away as Rome and Madison, Georgia. Lunch was served on tables decorated with fresh flowers and green table cloths. Clowns added to the festivity by distributing brightly-colored balloons and hats. The good time, laughter, and fellowship enjoyed by the company was summed up in a letter sent to the hospital later by a woman who had been a leukemia patient.

She wrote: "It amazed me that all the nurses were still working on that floor, because it's a tough place to be. These nurses are the most dedicated nurses in the world. They become a part of your family and you really rely on them." Of the party, she said, "If the nurses had not been there, you could have thrown all the decorations away. The fact that they are willing to go through all the trouble is what makes this reunion so special."

A male patient, given two months to live when Crawford Long doctors "started working on him" in 1983, said, "The Lord has been good to us. The reunion is a beautiful thing. People come together and realize what we've been through. This encourages you and lets others see how you're doing. It gives you hope." Grateful to his doctors, nurses and staff members, he said, "We're one family. Drs. Carr and Lokey, the nurses, maids—there's nothing like this bunch. We have to be thankful for them, they bring us through. How they all have as much patience as they do, I'll never know. They are really special people."

Another event that reunites staff members and former patients is the Annual Preemie Christmas Party. The fifth annual reunion saw a gathering of smiling parents, nursery workers and healthy youngsters who were born prematurely and often desperately ill.

The yearly party gives the nursery workers a chance to see the progress the preemies have made, and a chance to renew bonds forged during the time they cared for these special children.

The children, some still infants, were brought dressed in Christmas finery to meet Santa Claus who gave them dated, cross-stitched Christmas tree ornaments hand-made by the nursery staff. (Some of the children now have four ornaments from past holiday parties.) One couple brought their son, Oliver, all the way from

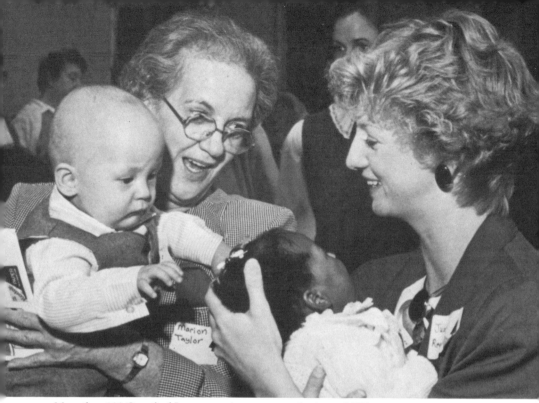

More than 100 Crawford Long preemie nursery graduates and 250 family members returned for the fifth annual preemie Christmas party. Wesley Reynolds (left) is held by Marion Taylor, administrative director of nursing, while Juanita Reynolds (right) cradles Katresea Wardley.

Chattanooga, Tennessee to celebrate. Other parents again expressed their gratitude for the care and concern extended to their babies.

Sherry Buchanan, Medical Social Worker, said, "This party provides us with gratification for what we've done in the past, hope for what we must do in the future. Each time we care for a desperately ill premature baby, we can remember how healthy and full of life these children are. It is easy to become emotionally involved and attached to these children and their families. It is thrilling to see them doing so well now."

CHEMOTHERAPY

In November 1985, Carol Hughes, RN, MSN, Oncology Clinical Nurse Coordinator, presented a seminar designed to enhance the quality of nursing care for the chemotherapy patient. This was sponsored by Crawford Long Hospital for the State of Georgia's "concerned medical people."

As a member of the American Cancer Society Professional Education Committee, she has been instrumental in planning oncology nursing seminars throughout the State. Her articles on nursing and cancer chemotherapy have appeared in the American Journal of Nursing and the Journal of the National Intravenous Association. She is also a co-author of *Cancer Therapy Administration Course*.

Miss Hughes developed the cancer chemotherapy program at Crawford Long. Her responsibilities include clinical and administrative management of the chemotherapy inpatient area and the oncology education for staff and students.

SOCIAL SERVICE

In spring 1987, Crawford Long's Social Service Department moved to expanded quarters on the third floor in the Nursing School Dormitory Building. This department employs six social workers with Suzanne Lomas as Director and Maple Caldwell as secretary-receptionist.

The social workers see between fifty and sixty new patients and their families per month, plus patients carried over from the month before.

Mrs. Lomas said, "An amazing amount of our work involves helping patient families cope with new situations, such as the reality of a hospital bed and commode in their living room. Sometimes the hardest job may be to locate a patient's family or friends in time of overwhelming [patient] need."

ANESTHESIOLOGY EXPANSION

In the early days of anesthesia, virtually any physician, nurse or occasional dentist would be called upon to administer an anesthetic to a patient about to undergo a surgical procedure. At the time Drs. Davis and Fischer opened their sanatorium, there were few trained anesthetists available and persons with varying experience and training assisted the surgeons. In later years, certified registered nurse anesthetists were added to the staff and in 1956, the first specially trained physician anesthesiologist joined the staff.

In the early 1970s, Dr. Carl Smith came to Crawford Long as Director of the Department of Anesthesiology. He has worked to develop a team approach to care for the patient undergoing anesthesia, and today, anesthesiologists, nurse anesthetists and physician's assistants work together caring for the patient before, during and after surgery.

As with other medical disciplines, anesthesia staff members often sub-specialize in areas such as pediatrics, cardiac surgery, pain control and other related fields, using their education and experience to enhance the total care of the patient.

Dr. Smith emphasized that the area of greatest potential growth in surgery and anesthesia for the future will be in the expanding treatment of patients on an outpatient basis. He noted that nearly 40% of surgical procedures may be performed in the outpatient setting and that development of the new outpatient surgery center at Crawford Long would place the hospital at the forefront of this movement.

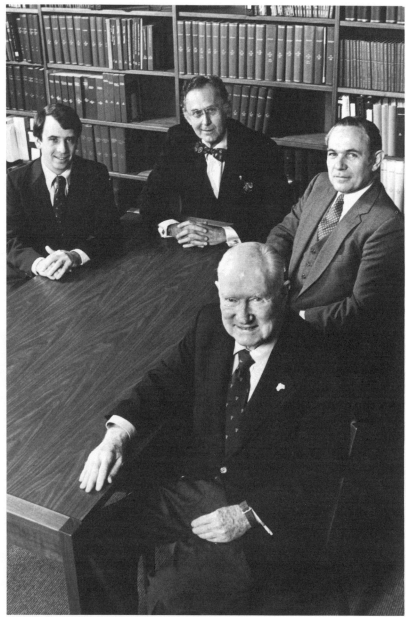

Clockwise, Mr. Ren Davis, Mr. W. Daniel Barker,
Mr. John Henry, and Dr. Wadley Glenn.

THE BUSINESS OF RUNNING A HOSPITAL

Before the discovery of anesthesia and x-rays, hospitals were places of pain and death. They were a last resort; some were called "pest houses." Rich and middle class people were treated at home, even for surgery. By the time Crawford Long Hospital was founded in 1908, medical standards had improved.

As the years passed, the public desire for top notch care at a low cost arose to pose a problem for hospitals and doctors.

A Montgomery Ward catalogue (1894-95) gives list prices of medical mortars and pestles at 15 cents, 20 cents, and 85 cents, depending on size. A "Dr. Forbes" bath and hot-bed thermometer was 48 cents. A spirit lamp sold for 40 cents. In 1968, one piece of equipment—an autoanalyzer—cost $40,000. In March of 1940, "Hospital Management" advertised bleached muslin surgeons' gowns in case lots of twenty-four dozen for $18.95. A charge of $70-75 a day was normal in 1971 in contrast to $55 per day in 1940.

The rising costs of hospital care concerned Mr. W. Dan Barker, Crawford Long Administrator, in 1968 when he said, "It's hard to put a price tag on hospital services." Mr. Barker likened the hospital to a city within a city, where a million meals a year were served. The Crawford Long medical staff of 530, plus 950 full-time employees and 223 part-time workers had to be paid. Educational programs for diploma nurses, intern and resident programs, medical and x-ray technology, inhalation therapy plus on-the-job training for nursing assistants added to the monetary costs.

In 1971, Mr. Barker stated, "This is our goal: To put ourselves out of business. If people would just go by the health habits they already know they would stay out of the hospital. It is just practicing common sense." He suggested that preventive medicine, including regular medical check-ups, and visits to the doctor when symptoms of ill health first appear, be used to prevent problems before they get out of hand.

"One of the things we'll be able to do in the new patient tower of Crawford Long is health education," Mr. Barker said in 1968. "In each floor we'll have educational conference rooms. If we can keep people from having to be admitted to hospitals we've done our best job." He mentioned other ways to save on hospital costs by taking advantage of community facilities, free chest x-ray examinations, diabetes tests or immunization by local health departments. He repeated that Crawford Long had a full-time nurse whose entire duty was to work with physicians and patients to try for earlier discharge. He mentioned such community resource groups as the Visiting Nurse Association or the Easter Seal Society.

Mr. Barker, in the March 1972 issue of "Atlanta Medicine" (a Medical Association of Atlanta bulletin) stated, "Most knowledgeable persons realize that hospitals have become the community's reservoir for specialized equipment, highly trained personnel and extensive physical facilities. The modern hospital is the vehicle through which most of the medical advances are integrated into improved delivery of health care."

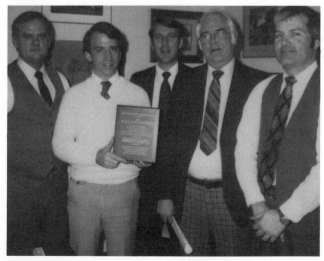

Cost Containment Committee, l-r: Gil Flournoy, Ren Davis, Robert Kimble, Greg Crook and Doug Bennett. Not shown is Mary Hart, RN.

In 1979, Crawford Long Hospital was recognized as the winner of the Pacer (Proven Application for Cost Effectiveness Reward) Contest for the best cost containment program in Georgia hospitals in 1979. The Pacer Award was established by the Blue Cross Plan and the Georgia Hospital Association to stimulate the development of cost accountability committees, to provide a monetary incentive reward for the most effective committees and to involve all hospital employees in cost containment.

Crawford Long did it again in 1982. Render Davis, Assistant Administrator, accepted the Cost Containment Award in the sixth annual presentation at the annual Georgia Hospital Association convention.

W. DANIEL BARKER

Mr. W. Daniel Barker came to Crawford Long Hospital in September 1960. Formerly the Crawford Long Administrator, he is now Director of Hospitals for the Robert W. Woodruff Health Sciences Center of Emory University. "The association with Crawford Long and being with Dr. Glenn for so many years," he said, "has been among the happiest times of my life."

Upon graduation from Emory in 1949, Mr. Barker took the position of Manager of the Business Office at Emory University. He held that position for a year. The next ten years he worked throughout the state in various hospital positions.

Mr. Barker recounted Atlanta's hospitals' history—"As we look at Crawford Long and its leaders, we see how many of the major hospitals in Atlanta have come together. Back in the early 1900s we had five major hospitals: Wesley Memorial which became Emory University Hospital when it moved to the Emory campus; Crawford Long Hospital (and interestingly enough Dr. Fischer was also on the initial Board of Trustees of the old Wesley Memorial Hospital when it was established on Auburn Avenue soon after the turn of the Century); Georgia Baptist Hospital in which my father, Mr. W. D. Barker, worked as administrator from 1931 until his death in 1946. My father and Dr. Fischer were instrumental in establishing the first Blue Cross Plan in this country in 1937 when it was known as the United Hospital Service Association.

"We also had St. Joseph's Infirmary, the oldest hospital in Atlanta, and Grady Memorial Hospital, which was our county and city hospital, and Piedmont Hospital which was one of the initial five private hospitals.

"Dr. Glenn's father was probably more instrumental than any other Georgia citizen in enacting the Hospital Authority Law of Georgia in 1941. For the first time, this officially separated the operation of hospitals owned by county or city government from the political structure that had been so common throughout the history of Georgia and the country as a whole.

"The Hospital Authority Law made it possible for institutions such as Grady Memorial Hospital to come into being, to have stronger financial base and to expand and be the major teaching facility we have today as far as the Emory affiliated hospitals are concerned.

"The camaraderie, the working together, the joint ventures of helping the total community rather than individual institutions was the name of the game back then rather than marketing, advertising and competition we see so much of today.

"Many refer to those days as the 'good old days' and from one standpoint, they were. We had common goals, we worked together. However, considering the new medical techniques now available, the care that is possible for us to provide, I'm not sure that any of us would really want to go back to 1908 or 1911 when the 'new' Crawford Long Hospital was built between the Peachtrees or even to the 1960s when I came back to Atlanta and to Crawford Long. Ninety percent of the things we do for patients now were unknown in 1908. And when 1990 and the year 2000 comes, we are going to see continuing of this scientific advancement in medicine.

"I think one of the things that makes Crawford Long different from most other institutions I have known is it recognizes that not only is there the quality of care so important but also the quality of service, the humane things that are done; the daily visits of Dr. Glenn and Mrs. Georgia Belle Martin to patients and now Dr. Ramos following Dr. Glenn's example . . . . Each community had certain health care needs that were a little different. So each hospital met them in different ways. One of the significant things about the Crawford Long Hospital is its understanding of those processes and its continued commitment to the community it serves.

"Crawford Long has always had an open staff. When there was a shortage of beds, many other hospitals in town closed their staffs to new physicians. This was never the case at Crawford Long.

"Both Dr. Fischer and Dr. Glenn felt limiting the number of

staff physicians had nothing to do with limiting the amount of sickness in the community. After all, that was the reason Crawford Long was established—to meet those needs.

"All institutions, particularly those as complex from a technical standpoint and from a social standpoint as a hospital, have problems. But problems assist us in finding new solutions, so from our standpoint, Crawford Long Memorial Hospital and its medical staff really has the best of both worlds. With a solid base of community support and a solid core of full-time faculty members, we are able to bring together the latest scientific advances in a way that makes them available to the community and to the mainstream of medicine almost instantaneously.

MONA TEMPLES

Mona Temples came to Crawford Long in 1963 to serve as Mr. Barker's Secretary. Almost from the beginning of her association with the hospital, she was interested in its history and was instrumental in saving many old documents, records, and memorabilia. She also helped on other projects, including the hospital cookbook and museum scrapbooks.

Mrs. Temples joined Mr. Barker at Emory University when he assumed his position as Emory's Director of Hospitals in 1984.

JOHN D. HENRY

Mr. John D. Henry became the Crawford Long Administrator and Chief Executive Officer in 1985. A close follower of his mentor Dr. Glenn, Mr. Henry became involved in growth for Crawford Long that has placed it in the forefront of Atlanta's hospitals. By the end of 1986, with the acquisition of the Doctors Memorial Hospital, Crawford Long was the second largest hospital in the city.

In summing up the year 1986, Mr. Henry recognized the hospital workers when he said, "Our employees make Crawford Long what it is today. Throughout the year, all of our departments were recognized individually for their dedication and commitment."

John Henry came to the hospital in August of 1963 as an Administrative Department employee. After being there a while, he said, "I can tell you in a few words why I stay at Crawford Long. I feel this hospital is making the most notable contribution to medical care service in Atlanta and because there isn't a finer person or better man to work with than Dr. Glenn."

Born in Atlanta, Mr. Henry attended Georgia Military Academy, Emory University, and the Medical College of Georgia before entering the United States Army where he was awarded the Army Commendation for Meritorious Service by the Army Medical Service School. He left the Army to go back to school at Georgia State College, where he studied hospital administration. Later he studied at Georgia Tech and attended a variety of seminars related to the ever changing and intricate demands of the administrative process of running a large community hospital.

An Associate Professor of Community Health at Emory University School of Medicine, he is Preceptor of Hospital Administration students from the University of Minnesota. He is on the Council of Finance for the AHA and Preceptor for Management Engineering from Georgia Tech.

He is a Fellow in the American College of Hospital Administrators and holds professional affiliations with the American Hospital Association, American Management Association, American Society for Hospital Engineering, American Society for Hospital Materials Management, Electrical Section of the National Fire Protection Association, Health Care Section of the National Fire Protection Association and Hospital Management Systems Society.

Mr. Henry and his wife, the former Barbara Jane Bailey, have two children, John D. Henry, Jr., M.D. and Karen, also an Emory graduate, who is an accountant.

NANCY YARN

Mrs. Nancy Yarn, retired Office Manager, has been a familiar person at Crawford Long Hospital for fifty years. She is still an active volunteer in the Crawford Long Museum.

Her introduction to working at Crawford Long came in 1921, when she worked for two weeks as a substitute cashier for a vacationing friend. When Mrs. Yarn learned Dr. Fischer's secretary, Mrs. Bailey, was planning a month's leave, she applied to act as temporary secretary.

Dr. Fischer told her the position required shorthand, and Mrs. Yarn assured him she could learn it before Mrs. Bailey left. With nothing more than four night school sessions in shorthand at

Central High before she married, Nancy Yarn tackled learning a full term's work in less than thirty days. "Dr. Fischer was very kind," she said. "Dictating very slowly rather than in his usual staccato style."

Mrs. Yarn returned to work at Crawford Long in 1937. "There were two of us in the Business Office then," said Mrs. Yarn. "Marguerite DeSmidt was Cashier and Medical Records Librarian and I handled the bookkeeping." Posting charges to patients' ledgers, making up bills, writing paychecks and keeping the check registers was all done by hand.

Nancy Yarn was appointed Office Manager to replace retiring Mrs. DeSmidt in 1953. At that time, Mrs. Yarn recalls, there was not in effect an accounts receivable program. She said, "We were on a cash basis." Bookkeeping eventually was done by machine and more people were added to the office.

With the installation of computers in 1967, a whole new field opened. "However," said Mrs. Yarn, "Changes were made without too much trauma due to cooperation of data processors Gil Flournoy and Jack Abbott. With them and Ada Roberts, the changeover was a breeze."

In a talk Mrs. Yarn presented to accountants in 1971, she named others who had contributed to the successful operation. They were Elizabeth Davis in Accounting; Ruth Goolsby and Louise Harvey in Insurance; Joy Rader in Payroll; Emily Cheek and Kay Tarleton in Cashiering; Louise Wallace in Accounts Receivable Control, Mary Jo Griffon Shiver in Credits; Myrtle Johnson in Admissions and Sara Quillian in Information.

When Mrs. Yarn marked thirty-five years of service to Crawford Long, she was chosen Employee of the Month. At that time, she described her affection for her work place and its people. "There is a feeling at this hospital," she said, "that is not the same anywhere else. It is a feeling the hospital cares about its employees."

She retired as Manager of the Business Office in 1971, but an article in the Northside News two years later reveals Mrs. Yarn didn't stay "retired" very long. The feature story said, "She worked on the building fund and later on a cookbook—a joint venture of the hospital and the Crawford Long Auxiliary members. At the suggestion of Mrs. Yarn, the cookbook was titled *Cooking With Love*, a play on the Crawford W. Long initials."

Mrs. Yarn published a book of poems, *Let it Rain*, in 1981 that is illustrated by her great grandson, Micheal Van Landingham.

Sold in the Auxiliary Gift Shop, the books' profits go back to the hospital. Poems written by Mrs. Yarn have appeared in The "Larynx" since it began publication in 1970. She also composed verses for hospital Christmas cards sent to employees and hospital friends.

She was married to the late Charles Yarn. Their children are Dr. Charles P. Yarn and Mrs. Barbara Rosenberg. She has six grand-children and one great grandson.

JANE HARRIMAN, MARLENE EUBANKS

Jane Harriman, Director of the Medical Records Department, recalls that department had only two people when she met with Dr. Glenn and Mrs. Eloise Hatcher in May of 1948. "I was to be in complete charge of the medical records and try to get things started," she said. "There was no master patient index file and records were stapled together as they came down from the floors." Her duties included charge of the medical library which contained, in addition to a thousand medical books, copies of the fifty to sixty medical journals received each month. Anyone employed by the hospital had access to the library.

By the end of Mrs. Harriman's first year of work at Crawford Long, a file clerk was hired and the records department moved to more spacious quarters. By 1957, the Medical Records Department employed twelve people and was housed in a still larger area. When the new Peachtree Building opened in 1973, the records department moved there, but still has twelve employees despite an increasing workload and computerization.

Mrs. Marlene Eubanks, assistant to Mrs. Harriman since 1961, now works with most of the coders entering data which "has evolved into a good system, relieving a lot of the earlier manual work." Mrs. Eubanks became director of the department following Mrs. Harriman's retirement in 1985.

ADA ROBERTS

When Ada Roberts reported for work in the Business Office of Crawford Long Hospital on August 21, 1951, it was located just off the old Linden Avenue lobby. Then there was one fairly large office and three private offices and a glassed-in cashier's unit stretch-ing across the front of the office.

Mrs. Roberts said of that modest set-up compared with

today's extensive operation, "There was an office manager and one assistant to delegate work duties, supervise and pitch in and work with the other eight to ten employees. So small was the operation in the early 1950s, current and outstanding patient files were stored in one file cabinet.

"In 1966, the wonderful age of the computer began at Crawford Long when accounts receivables were computerized. Office work was revolutionized. Payroll records went on computer and other material was added each year thereafter. It was amazing to see work that was completed in a week before now produced in thirty to forty-five minutes," said Mrs. Roberts.

After thirty-five years of service, Mrs. Roberts retired.

LOIS SMITH

Before 1964, outpatient accounts were handled by "whoever had a few minutes to spare." That year, Lois Smith recalls, the Outpatient Department was set up to combine outpatient collection with that of the Emergency Room patients. The first office was a desk in the hall. Mrs. Smith opened the office and handled the department for two years before Mrs. Janice Lussardi was added to take care of Medicare and Medicaid.

Then an ambulance entrance information and admissions came under the Outpatients Accounts Department. Patients' mail was routed through it too. Auxiliary volunteers, working five days a week, helped alleviate the workload.

"Today," Mrs. Smith said, "We have grown from that one desk in the hall to five full-time employees, one part-time worker and two men who alternate night work from 7 p.m.-7 a.m."

Mrs. Smith remembers "minor miracles" performed by Emergency Department workers. Some incidents were amusing.

For example, she recalls a frantic telephone call that alerted the emergency crew to meet a "very sick patient being brought in for treatment." The "patient" proved to be an ailing dog.

"We kept a straight face and found a vet for the dog," said Mrs. Smith with a grin.

DATA PROCESSING

When Gilbert Flournoy, Director of Data Processing, came

to Crawford Long Hospital April 4, 1966, no automation existed. Computer equipment was one IBM 1440. Mr. Flournoy's first office was tucked away in a pantry of the Woodruff Building. Above his desk were cabinets that once held linen.

Flournoy said, "Coming into the hospital environment was a totally new experience for me. It was like coming into a big happy family. Everyone connected with Data Processing was always willing to lend a helping hand."

Flournoy's first task was to install a patient billing system on the computer with the aid of an IBM engineer. The system was in place in December 1966. Personnel from the Business Office were trained to operate the keypunch machines and the computer.

In the latter part of 1966, Ann Edwards was hired as an assistant. Since that time, she has advanced to become Operations Manager.

"In January of 1967," Flournoy said, "Jack Abbott, now Assistant Director of Data Processing, came with us as a programmer." He began development of a medical records system.

Flournoy said, "To begin with, Dr. Glenn was reluctant to bring a computer into the system but with the achieved success, he became one of its strongest supporters. His periodic visits to Data Processing along with a new story or joke were always welcomed and enjoyed."

In December of 1968, Owen Davidson joined the staff as a programmer helping to put new applications on the computer. He later became Systems and Programming Manager.

Mr. Gilbert Flournoy and Mr. Jack Abbott of Data Processing.

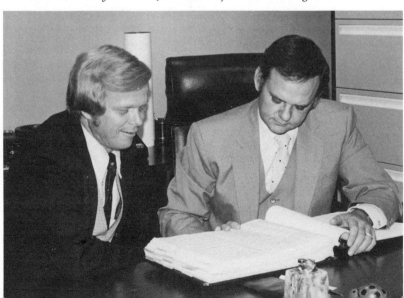

To name all who have contributed to the success of the Data Processing Department would "require a book in itself," according to Mr. Flournoy. "With most of the departments and nursing units connected to the computers, we are doing work for almost every area in the hospital. Our staff has grown from myself in 1966 to one of forty-two persons.

"We are now into a new phase of growth with joint development in applications occurring between Crawford Long Hospital and Emory University Hospital."

GREGORY CROOK

Gregory M. Crook, Assistant Administrator and Chief Financial Officer, with his staff, is responsible for patient admission and discharge. Crook said, "Getting proper information from incoming patients, processing it adequately in the Business Office and having correct information as far as diagnosis is concerned in Medical Records is vitally pertinent to file claims." His goal is to speed it up and make the process as smooth as possible for the patient.

Mr. Crook, a native of Alabama, came to Crawford Long Hospital in 1969 after several years' work in Florida hospitals. Medical Records and the Business Office, Social Services and Utilization Review and Medical Transcription now all come under his jurisdiction.

"We have so many new things now," he said. "Such as HMO [Health Maintenance Organization] and PROs [Preferred Provider Organization]. Here we deal with the purchaser of services directly. We try to conserve costs. Patients have paid for care. We try to provide it."

JOSEPH T. MASSEY, JR.

Joseph T. Massey, Jr., Communication Consultant for Crawford Long, likes to tell his interest in communications began when he was nine years old. Then he worked at the switchboard of his father's Macon, Georgia motel.

As a Georgia Tech student in 1969, he applied for part-time work as a switchboard operator—then thought of as a woman's occupation. Mrs. Jeanette Tyson, Chief Operator, let him demonstrate his skill. He was hired.

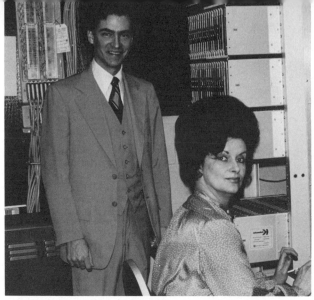

*Mr. Joseph T. Massey, Jr. and Ms. Carolyn Anglin
in the 1979 equipment room.*

As a part of his design project in Industrial Engineering at Georgia Tech, Massey approached Mr. Dan Barker for permission to examine the hospital telephone bills to see if there could be a reduction in billing. His analysis revealed the hospital could save approximately $10,000 a year by converting to a flat-rate service at a nominal conversion fee.

Mr. Massey was asked to write specifications for the telephone system for the Peachtree Tower when it was in the planning stage in 1970. He said, "I wrote the specification as part of my project in industrial engineering and Southern Bell agreed with Western Electric to build the telephone system tailored to my specifications."

Of his career at Crawford Long Hospital, Mr. Massey said, "I wouldn't trade the years I've been here for anything else in the world."

GIRIJA VIJAY

Mrs. Girija Vijay, Director of Crawford Long Medical Library, received her Masters degree from Atlanta University Library School where she worked for three years at the School of Library Service. She received certification in medical librarianship from Emory University in 1971.

When Mrs. Vijay began her work at Crawford Long August 8, 1971, the library was under the School of Nursing Director, Ann Stroud.

During her fifteen years at the library, it was rated as "The Best Hospital Library in Georgia" by the Southeastern Medical Library Program. Mark Hodges, director of the program, brought twenty librarians to review the Crawford Long Library as a sample of a good hospital library.

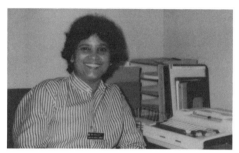

Mrs. Girija Vijay, Director of Crawford Long Medical Library.

Mrs. Vijay said, "We are a member of the Emory Medical Television Network since its inception and we have an available list of media collection. We are the only library with two professional librarians since 1974."

The library now has six staff members and is open seven days a week, welcoming physicians, nurses and employees.

FREDA MOSS

Freda Moss is Administrator of the Jesse Parker Williams Hospital. "This is a job that perhaps requires a woman," she said, "in that you have only women and children including boys under twelve years of age as patients. There has always been a woman administrator here ever since the beginning of the hospital." Mrs. Moss came to work at Jesse Parker Williams December 8, 1975.

A soft-voiced, compassionate woman, Mrs. Moss is the person who makes the decisions on payment of bills. She said, "I feel humble that the Trustees allow me to make these decisions. For an example—Mary Jones comes in without money or any insurance. She has no family support or a job; yet she gets the same treatment as any paying patient. It is my responsibility to decide if she can or cannot pay her bill. It's a genuine pleasure to help those who try. I feel honored that I've been put in a position to help people."

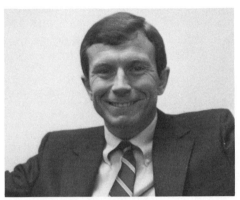

Mr. Mendel Bouknight, Director
of the Office of Development.

MENDAL BOUKNIGHT

Mendal Bouknight, Director of the Office of Development, is part of a new approach in publicizing what Crawford Long Hospital has to offer its patients and the community.

A native of South Carolina, he graduated from Clemson University, and earned a Masters degree at the University of Georgia School of Journalism. He spent three years as Alumni Program Director for the Alumni Relations Office at Emory University.

When he came to Crawford Long, he said, "There was in place a wealth of talent and services which could be communicated to the public." He established a new publication, *Viewpoint*, to reach former patients and friends of the hospital. He gave the in-house publication the "Larynx" a new look.

"We have the facilities, the personnel and the technology," he said. "Crawford Long has long been recognized as an outstanding hospital when the population was more centrally located and prior to the development of the suburban areas. Now there is the opportunity to make it known as a regional center for service."

NUTRITION SERVICES

James Greenhill, Director of Nutrition Services, said of his department, "The food operation is the result of the Nutrition Services management team. Assisting him are Barbara Rubino, RD,

Associate Director, and Lynn Moore, RD, Assistant Director.

Ruefully Mr. Greenhill said, "Every person who eats here at Crawford Long judges us at every meal according to his or her own special tastes and preferences. We serve 3,000 meals a day."

Among food items used in a regular month of meal preparation are 3,200 pounds of chicken, 1,200 pounds of bacon, 1,400 turkey breasts, 1,440 pounds of green beans, and 3,000 pounds of french fries; 22,000 four-ounce servings of orange juice are consumed in a month. The hospital spends $1.3 million a year on food and shares a purchasing program with Emory and Egleston Hospitals.

Mr. Greenhill is a University of Virginia graduate, and was a training sergeant in the United States Army Medical Corps. He came to Crawford Long following the retirement of longtime director, Sibyl Short. Mrs. Short joined the staff in 1964 and oversaw the major renovation of the kitchen and the cafeteria in 1980.

Mrs. Rubino, a graduate of Berry College with a degree in Institutional Management, oversees patient service including patient meal service and clinical dietetics.

Miss Moore, a graduate of the University of Alabama, is responsible for non-patient services—cafeteria, supply ordering, and inventory control.

All patients are screened by the clinical dietary staff to determine nutritional needs. Patients are followed up by nutrition counseling before they go home. Those who need to follow a special diet can call back for help or advice.

TELECOMMUNICATION SERVICE

The Crawford Long Telecommunication Department records 10,000 incoming calls a day, about 10,000 outgoing calls and 10,000 internal calls in an average business day. With these there are about 3,000 long distance calls for the entire network consisting of Crawford Long, Emory, Grady, and Egleston Hospitals and the Emory Clinic.

With transmitters on Stone and Sweat Mountains, the new digital beeper paging system has a swifter contact process with a range of sixty to eighty miles allowing doctors to keep in close communication with patient needs.

Carolyn Anglin, Telecommunication Director, said, "Today's telephone operators have long since outgrown Lily Tomlin's character 'Ernestine,' the simple-minded operator. They must know how to handle advanced and complicated computers."

Operators are trained to be pleasant to all callers and to keep calm in frightening situations, such as a distraught woman calling to say her child has swallowed poison. The operator stays on the line with her until she knows help has come, an ambulance is summoned or a call made to the Grady Poison Control Unit. "That has to do with personalized service that not all hospitals have. We think this is more important than saving dollars and cents."

MEDICAL TRANSCRIPTION

The Medical Transcription Department with Mrs. Mary Ann Hughey as Director and Mrs. Cheryl Peacock as Assistant Director now has eleven employees, eight full-time and three part-time workers.

In the hospital's early years, the Medical Transcription Department had only one transcriber, Miss Mattie Clyde Windham, who was employed at Crawford Long Hospital for 35 years. As the department enlarged, other transcribers were hired.

Mrs. Hughey said, "Transcriptionists must be capable of transcribing reports from almost every field of medicine—histories, physicals, operative notes, consultations and discharge summaries. It is a demanding and stressful job."

Mrs. Hughey came to Crawford Long as an intern in October of 1974 as part of her secretarial school training. She decided to stay on when she found her work so satisfying. She said, "the main reason I stayed was because I love working at Crawford Long and the people I work with."

Mrs. Hughey said, "In the past, a good turnaround time for histories, physicals and consultations was twenty-four hours; for operative notes, forty-eight hours and discharge summaries, five to seven days. That time has been virtually cut in half."

ROBERT J. BACHMAN

Robert J. Bachman's association with Crawford Long Hospital began in August 1975, when he started as Director of the Respiratory Therapy Department.

Mr. Bachman has served as Assistant Administrator for Patient Services since 1984. Mr. Bachman noted the long special tradition the hospital has played in providing health care to the Atlanta community. He said, "Crawford Long is like one large family with people helping people."

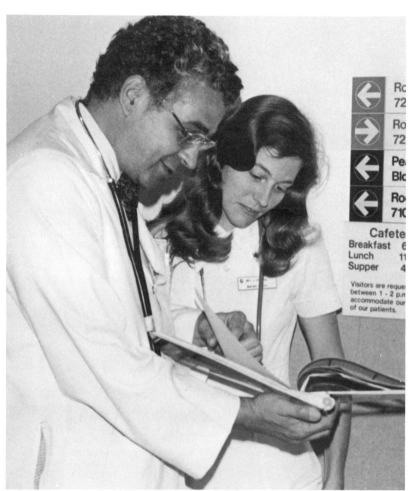

Dr. Harold Ramos speaks with a nurse.

MEDICAL PERSONNEL
STORIES

$\mathcal{T}$hroughout this book, mention is made of physicians, nurses and related workers at Crawford Long Hospital. This chapter highlights many of the long-time medical personnel workers. Hospital files hold a long list of young doctors who have walked the halls of the hospital as they sharpened the skills they learned in medical schools. The Crawford Long Nursing School has graduated hundreds of nurses. Among the thousands of Crawford Long patients, from aging senators to the new mothers, there exists a deep affection and gratitude for individual care and concern from those they always mention as "my doctor" or "my nurse."

DR. HAROLD RAMOS

Dr. Harold Ramos, Medical Director of Crawford Long Hospital, was born in Atlanta and schooled at Boys High School before he went to Johns Hopkins College. He matriculated there with a scholarship arranged for him by Dr. Edgar Paullin, who had been President Franklin Roosevelt's physician.

His education was interrupted by the death of his father, but later he received his medical training at the Medical College of Georgia. After graduation, Dr. Ramos donned a service uniform and, while on duty, did his residency at the Walter Reed Hospital in Washington, D.C. This was followed by a tour of duty with the United States Air Force in Wiesbaden, Germany. He returned to the States to take up an assignment at Keesler Air Force Base in Mississippi where he started a House Staff and Medical Service Program. There he was Chief of Medical Service.

Upon completion of his military stint, while visiting a service friend, Dr. Garland Herndon in Atlanta, he had his first interview in October 1962. In December, he was offered a place on the House Staff Training Program at Crawford Long. For the next ten years, plans were made, changed, and reformulated; eventually, the Emory Affiliated Training Program took shape and buildings were completed.

Dr. Ramos was appointed Crawford Long Hospital Medical Director on unanimous vote of the Woodruff Health Sciences Center Board, following the death of Dr. Glenn.

DR. DUDLEY KING

Dr. Dudley King, former Chief Radiologist at Crawford Long, came to work there April 1, 1949. Dr. King recalls being intrigued by Dr. Glenn's decided Southern accent coming through to him in a telephone call in the fall of 1948. Within days, he received a letter offering him employment in the X-ray Department. Dr. William Lake, then department head, had suffered a heart attack. John Dudley King, a native Texan, graduated from the University of Texas and received his medical degree there as well. He did his internship and three years residency in radiology at Cleveland Metropolitan Hospital.

In 1974, Michele Vizzini and Joy Pooran added luster to the reputation of the Crawford Long X-ray Department.

When they were students in the X-ray Technology Training Program, Miss Vizzini won first place in the 245th Meeting of the Georgia Society of Technologists in Augusta, Georgia. Mrs. Pooran was fourth place.

"When I first came to the hospital," Dr. King said, "the statement was made to me by an obstetrician that every third or fourth person you pass on an Atlanta street was born at Crawford Long Hospital. At that time, the Obstetrical Service was the biggest service at the hospital. With the exception of Grady Hospital, we delivered more babies here than any hospital in the Southeast."

"If I had it to do all over again, I would certainly choose Crawford Long Hospital. It is with a great deal of pleasure I look back over the years I have been here. It has been a tremendous experience!"

Dr. King retired in August 1986.

DR. J. RONALD STEPHENS

Dr. J. Ronald Stephens' whole life has been touched by Crawford Long Hospital. He was born November 1, 1941 at Crawford Long, delivered by Dr. Harry Ridley. "The first person who picked me up from Dr. Ridley," he said, "was Mrs. Ward, who carried me from the delivery room to let my father hold me."

His father, Crawford Long chief engineer from 1944 until his death in 1972, often brought young "Ron" to work with him. When the boy was fifteen years old, he joined his dad working at Crawford Long. During the summer and Christmas holidays, he worked in the supply room under the direction of Mrs. Ford. While a student at Emory University, he worked part-time in the Recovery Room; during his later college days he was employed in the Operating Room as a technician.

After graduation from Emory in 1966 with a BA degree, Stephens joined the United States Navy. Upon discharge, he returned to Crawford Long to work as an Operating Room technician and took additional courses at Georgia State University.

In 1968, he entered the Medical College of Georgia in Augusta. Between his first and second year he worked with Dr. Jim Olley as an extern in the Pathology Department. He graduated from medical school in 1972. After internship and residency in surgery at the Medical College of Georgia, Dr. Stephens stayed on there as a full-time associate professor of surgery for a year.

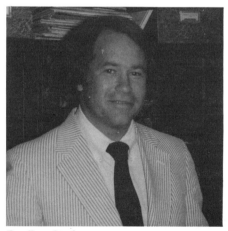

Dr. Ron Stephens

But Crawford Long and Atlanta called him back. "Working at Crawford Long has not merely been a position of employment but a family. The hospital paid for the education that led me to attend medical school and become a physician."

Dr. Stephens was named Crawford Long's Chief of Surgery on July 1, 1986, when Dr. Jesse W. Veatch retired.

DR. ALBERT L. EVANS

Dr. Albert L. Evans served in the United States Army in World War II. He went into the Army after his internship at Grady Hospital, six months before Pearl Harbor. His first duty was at Lawson General Hospital in Atlanta where he served two years. Later, as a result of action in the Battle of the Bulge, he was decorated.

Albert Evans, born in Sandersville, Georgia, received his education at Mercer University in Macon, earned an MD degree at Emory University Medical School. He entered private practice of general surgery, became associated with Dr. Olin Cofer and worked with him many years.

Dr. Evans and his wife have a happy memory of a day spent at Flowerland. Dr. Evans recalls Dr. Fischer enjoyed pointing out the many species of unusual flowers that made his gardens so famous.

Dr. Evans enjoys his profession: "Despite hard work and heartaches at times, the practice of medicine is the most satisfying work a young man could choose for his life's work."

DR. C. DOYLE HAYNES

Dr. C. Doyle Haynes came to Crawford Long in the fall of 1986 when he left his private practice in Opelika, Alabama. A graduate of Auburn University, Dr. Haynes received his medical degree from the Emory University School of Medicine.

He was a fellow of the American College of Surgeons, Diplomate of the American Board of Surgery and a fellow of the American College of Angiology. He was past president of the Alabama Chapter of the American College of Surgeons. Named Best Clinical Professor in the Emory University School of Medicine, he was professor of Surgery at the Emory School of Medicine since 1966 and was a member of the Emory Clinic. He was the recipient of the National

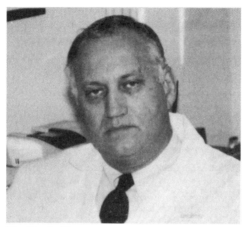

Dr. Doyle Haynes

Merit Award in Trauma from the American College of Surgeons in 1984. He also served the United States Air Force. Dr. Haynes died of a heart attack April 26, 1987.

Mr. John D. Henry had praise for Dr. Haynes and his work. He said, "We were fortunate to have a man of Dr. Haynes' caliber at Crawford Long Hospital. He brought the talents of a skilled surgeon and strong leadership qualities to our surgical staff, which were examples to all of us at the hospital. We are saddened by his death."

Dr. Charles Hatcher, Jr., Vice-president for Health Affairs and Director of The Robert W. Woodruff Health Sciences Center of Emory University, said of Dr. Haynes, "The medical profession has lost a truly outstanding individual."

A memorial service was held for Dr. Haynes in the Glenn Building Auditorium on April 28, 1987. Dr. Haynes is survived by his wife, Dena Hugley Hayes; two daughters, Mrs. Dallis Haynes Howard and Mrs. Lisa Haynes Horsely; and a son, Columbus Doyle Haynes, Jr.; his mother, Beulah Haynes and two sisters, Rowena Haynes Bolland and Ann Haynes Waid.

DR. GEORGE A. WILLIAMS

Dr. George Williams, a 1924 graduate of Emory University School of Medicine, devoted his long and distinguished career to the care and of mothers and their babies at Crawford Long. Dr. Williams was a pioneer in emphasizing the importance of prenatal care and was selected one of the first Fellows of the American College of Obstetrics and Gynecology.

The number of children who have come into this world under his skillful hands totals in the thousands. The Labor and Delivery Suite at Crawford Long is named in his honor.

GEORGIA BELLE MARTIN, RN

Georgia Belle Hearn Martin's association with Crawford Long Hospital began more than forty-five years ago when she was a young girl eager to become a nurse. A graduate of the Tallulah Falls School in North Georgia, she was working as a governess for an Atlanta family when she met with Dr. Fischer. Aware of her financial situation, Dr. Fischer arranged for her to receive nurse's training

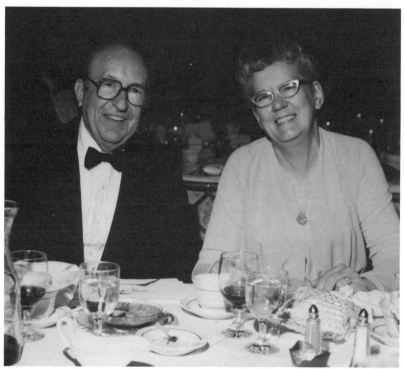

Mr. Shirley Martin and Mrs. Georgia Belle Martin

with uniforms and all the necessities for her schooling, with repayment to be made after she graduated.

Upon her graduation in 1944, she became Acting Director of the Nursing Service and served in that capacity until 1958, when she became Dr. Glenn's Executive Assistant.

It was Mrs. Martin who succeeded in getting a day care nursery for the children of working nurses, and she was there when the recovery room program was established, the program that completely changed post-operative care everywhere.

Mrs. Alice Martin, who was Supervisor of the Operating Room when Georgia Belle Martin came in as student, said, "She has been a mainstay in this hospital since she came."

Mrs. Nancy Yarn also had words of praise for Mrs. Martin's dependability. She said, "If Georgia Belle said she would do it, she did it. She got things done."

Dr. Harold Ramos, Medical Director, was quoted as saying, "Her retirement will leave a void that we will find difficult to fill.

"She cut through red tape. Because she made everything run so smoothly, people sometime did not realize how much work went into the process."

Mr. John Henry said, "We are all grateful for all she has given Crawford Long Hospital and to those of us here who worked with her."

The Crawford Long family turned out for Mrs. Martin's retirement party. Mr. Henry, recalling her long association with Crawford Long that made it her second home, said, "Like home, the door to Crawford Long will always be open."

ALICE MARTIN, RN

When Alice Martin came to work at Crawford Long Hospital on April 20, 1942, she worked a 7 p.m.-7 a.m. shift for six weeks straight as Assistant Operating Room Supervisor. Miss Vera Bowen was the OR Supervisor, and she and other Crawford Long nurses were preparing to join the Emory Unit #43 for overseas duty. When Miss Bowen left, Mrs. Martin worked with Ila Alexander, the new OR Supervisor, until February of 1943 when she became the supervisor.

"We prepared all supplies used in OR and in the rest of the hospital, she remembers. "This included sharpening needles, patching gloves, making fluffs from washed sponges and rolling bandages. In spite of what now seems primitive conditions, we did not have hospital-acquired infections."

During World War II, Crawford Long carried the surgical load for the entire city. It was necessary to staff the OR twenty-four hours a day, seven days a week. "Our anesthesiologist was Dr. Charles E. Lawrence. We had three staff nurse anesthetists and three part-time anesthetists who were doctors' wives."

After twelve years as OR Supervisor, Mrs. Martin transferred to Nursing Service where she conducted orientation classes for nursing assistants and other Nursing Service personnel. She later assisted Katherine Pope, the Nursing Service Director.

"Then," said Mrs. Martin, "After my thirty years in Nursing Service, Mr. Dan Barker, Hospital Administrator, asked me to organize and manage a credit union. This I did until my retirement November 1,1985, thirteen and a half years later." She now devotes time to working in the Auxiliary Gift Shop and guides visitors in the Crawford Long Museum.

Mr. Barker presents Alice Martin
with a gift for her 40 years of service.

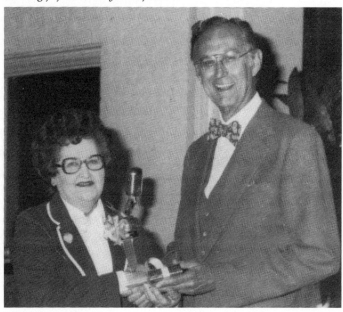

GLENDORA ROBINSON, RN

Glendora Robinson worked for twenty years at Crawford Long Hospital. A nurse who served in the United States Army, she earned a masters degree at Emory University. Her career at Crawford Long was spent as an instructor in Medical-Surgical Nursing and Trends in Nursing.

Mr. Henry presents a gift to Miss Ruth Duncan for her years of service to the hospital.

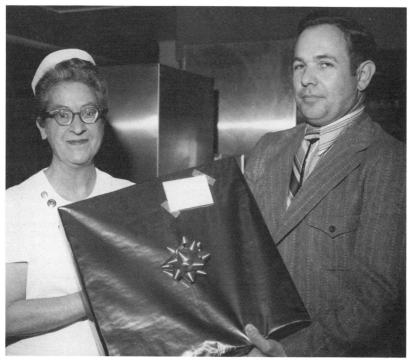

RUTH DUNCAN, RN

Ruth Duncan, RN, graduated from Davis-Fischer Sanatorium in 1931 with a Davis-Fischer pin and a diploma that reads Crawford Long Hospital. She was the head nurse on 3-B for many years. In 1972, Mr. Henry presented her a silver tray in recognition of her thirty-five years of devoted work at Crawford Long Hospital.

NADINE RUBIN, RN

The night nurse or "night owl" is a special person to doctors and patients alike. Nadine Rubin, a 1953 Crawford Long Nursing School graduate, worked on the night shift (11 p.m.-7 p.m.) for seventeen years. "Patients need a nurse more at night," Mrs. Rubin said. "Many nurses feel they can get closer to a patient, can do more for the really sick ones at night."

HARRIET WARD, RN

Harriet Ward, a Crawford Long Nursing School graduate, decided to work there despite a daily eighteen mile drive from Jonesboro because, she said, "It's like home to me."

When the fifteen bed Intermediate Intensive Coronary Care Unit opened in 1961, she became its head nurse. In a 1971 issue of the "Larynx," she gave her philosophy of how best to treat the seriously ill patients in her care. She said, "Have knowledge—and a sense of humor. Make the patient feel like a person."

MARY REISWEBER, RN

Mary Reisweber, RN, began an Employee Health Program in July 1976. She supervised pre-employment physicals and met with regular employees for their once-a-year check-up on the anniversary of their employment, or when they had a health-related problem.

Mrs. Reisweber's work in Personnel began with a corner desk and one file drawer. In 1976, her office included an examination area and ten file drawers. By 1984, her work included pap smear clinics and blood drives held three times a year, a working relation with the Environmental Health Committee, immunization procedures, and aerobics classes for employees.

ELSIE REEVES, RN

Elsie Reeves, RN, came to Crawford Long for an appendectomy and spent twenty-three days in Jesse Parker Williams when she was sixteen years old. It was then she made up her mind to become a nurse.

Upon graduation from high school, she worked as a nurse's aide in The Williams Hospital and then she became a Crawford Long student nurse, graduated and went to work at Jesse Parker Williams.

JEAN WATSON, RN, BS

Jean Watson, a Crawford Long graduate with a BS degree from Georgia State University, said in 1971, "I've seen duty on every floor and in every department of the hospital." Twenty-seven years after the Crawford Long Recovery Room was established as the first in Atlanta, Miss Watson, as its head nurse, was proud of its accomplishments—"a coordination of careful monitoring of patients in the most efficient and beneficial way for all."

MARGARET FOWLER, RN

Another Crawford Long Nursing School graduate who worked at Crawford Long Hospital for many years was Margaret Fowler, Operating Room Supervisor.

In 1971 she was quoted in the "Larynx" as saying, "I was born and reared at Crawford Long. I've had forty years at its bed-sides."

To ease the anxiety of a family worrying and waiting out an operation on a loved one, Mrs. Fowler saw to it someone phoned.a progress report from the operating room. "We stress the fact that every patient belongs to somebody," she said.

From 1974 until her retirement in 1987, Mrs. Fowler served as nurse director of the hospital's utilization program.

RUBYE DAVID, RN

Rubye David was employed by Crawford Long in September of 1943 to assist surgeons during operations. She was a close assistant, taking the place of young doctors who were away in war-time service. After the war, she left Crawford Long to work in the office of Dr. Harry Ridley, and then she was an instructor at the Atlanta Dental College, which became the Emory Dental School.

In 1954, she returned to Crawford Long to work as a scrub nurse for Dr. Glenn and for other surgeons. In 1974, she became

Operating Room Supervisor and served in that capacity until her retirement in 1985.

LOUISE DAWKINS, RN, and CLARA MAHONEY, RN

Louise Dawkins and Clara Mahoney, nurse anesthetists, retired in March 1972. They were presented gifts in recognition of twenty-five years of service to Crawford Long Hospital.

Miss Mahoney trained at Crawford Long Nursing School and was an Army nurse in World War II with the rank of captain.

RALPH JENKINS

Ralph Jenkins came to work in the Crawford Long X-ray Department in 1958 and worked there until illness forced retirement.

His wife, Mattie Jean, has worked for Dr. Glenn and Mrs. Georgia Belle Martin and now works for Dr. Ramos. Mr. Jenkins said, "I am very proud of her and the work she does at the hospital."

NUCLEAR MEDICINE

Nuclear medicine, considered a new but expanding field in 1971, was headed by Dr. Ernest G. Smith. At the time, he was one of five physicians in Georgia devoting full time to nuclear medicine. Dr. Smith, who was on the staff of the Emory University School of Medicine, came to Crawford Long Hospital in 1969. Dr. Scheidt now serves as director of the department, following Dr. Smith's retirement.

Founded in 1964, the Nuclear Medicine Department provided physicians with modern techniques for diagnosing and treating patients with brain, thyroid gland, lung, kidney, liver, spleen, pancreas, bone, and other disorders.

Nuclear medicine uses radioactive materials to help diagnose and treat a wide variety of diseases and disorders. For emission scanning, the patient is given a radioactive compound which travels through the body giving off gamma rays (invisible radiation) that tell how the drug travels and how long it takes to reach the part of the body being studied. Special equipment detects the gamma rays and shows them on a TV screen. The results are interpreted by a specialist who, in turn, advises the patient's regular doctor.

The six most widely used tests are brain and bone scans, thyroid uptakes and scans, lung and liver scans and cardiac imaging. Most procedures are expensive because they require highly skilled professionals, intricate equipment, and elaborate safety measures.

The nuclear medicine team consists of a nuclear medicine physician, a nuclear medicine technologist, and a nuclear medicine physicist.

KATHERINE POPE, RN, BSN

Katherine Pope, Assistant Administrator for Nursing Service, is an integral part of the story of the Crawford Long Nursing School. Miss Pope came to Crawford Long in April 1958 as a part-time faculty member. In September of 1958, she became Acting Director of Nursing Service.

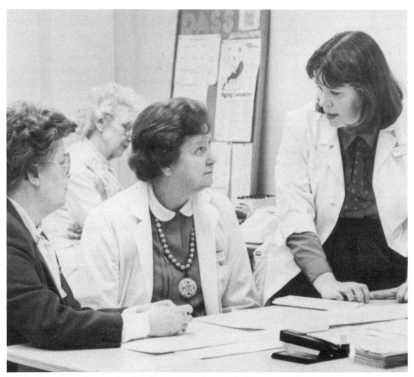

Katherine Pope (center) with Joyce Horsley and Margaret Anderson

She came from Grady Memorial Hospital where she cared for polio victims when many patients were kept alive in iron lungs. There Miss Pope met Mrs. Macie Stephens, then Director of Nursing Service at Crawford Long. Mrs. Stephens was visiting a Crawford Long student who was a patient at Grady Hospital. The two nurses became friends, and it was through this contact Miss Pope came to Crawford Long.

Miss Pope's affection for Crawford Long is evident. She said, "It is a family community. If you are a member of the Crawford Long Hospital employee group, you are a member of the family. This hospital, as a family, has served this city and its citizens.

"At Christmas time and special occasions, if a former employee is back in the community, they still came back, referring to Crawford Long as 'home.' Recently Annette Brianan, a Crawford Long graduate who was honored by the Georgia Nurses Association came by. We have visitors who say to the staff, proudly, 'I was born here.' I feel a part of that family—an exciting experience."

In 1987, Katherine Pope was recognized for her volunteer work with Downtown Atlanta Senior Services (DASS), a support organization for the in-town elderly. She received the highest honor awarded volunteers at the annual DASS recognition luncheon.

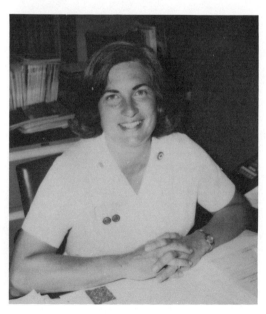

Mary Hart, RN, Associate Director Nursing Service.

MARY G. HART, RN, BS

Mary G. Hart, RN, BS, Associate Director, Nursing Service, has devoted twenty-two years to Crawford Long Hospital going back to her student days at the hospital's School of Nursing.

She started her nursing career as a staff nurse, became head nurse in the Orthopedics and Neuro and Thoracic Departments in January 1966. From there she became Supervisor of the Nursing Service. She advanced to Associate Director in February 1982.

Mrs. Hart has words of praise for Katherine Pope, the Assistant Administrator for Nursing, saying, "I have worked under the direction of Katherine Pope most of my twenty-two years at the hospital. She has been very active at both the national and local levels in nursing and shares an outstanding reputation among her colleagues."

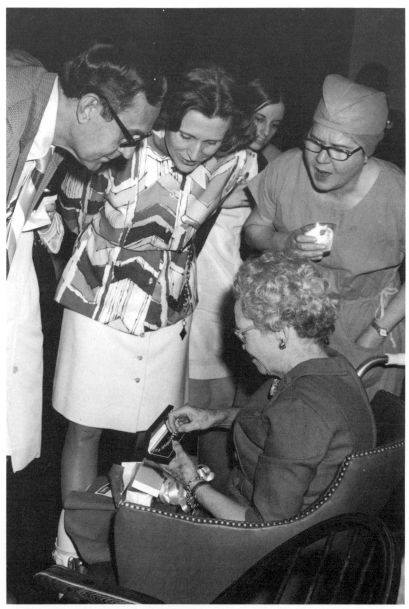

Mr. W. Daniel Barker, Miss Betty Dailey
and Miss Christine Cassels (left to right)
admire a charm bracelet given to Miss Mahoney ·(seated).

CHAPTER FIFTEEN

LONGTIME EMPLOYEE STORIES

A Hospital Is Not Built of Stone

A hospital is not really built
of steel and masonry
It's built of service given
By folks like you and me.
It's built up—not by concrete walls
And floors of marble tile
But by a sincere wish to help.
A gentle hand, a smile
That drives back all that cold expanse
Of huge and lonely space
And gives it warmth and spirit—
A proper healing place!
No, a hospital is not really built
Just of steel and masonry
It is built of love and caring
By folks like you and me!

—Nancy Yarn

The "Larynx" is the hospital publication that keeps the Crawford Long family informed. Dr. Glenn's columns through the years gave encouragement. Department progress articles let workers on the night shift know what was going on during the day; those working in the kitchen learned of progress in medicine.

Long-time workers were chosen to be featured in Larynx pages. Following are excerpts from "Larynx" stories of loyal and dedicated workers who were featured during the course of the years.

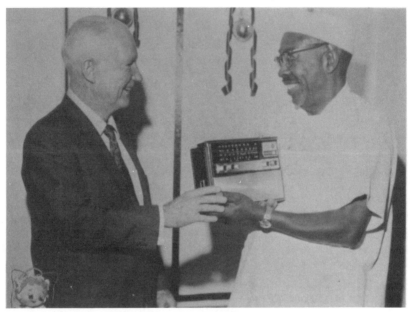

Mr. James Tuggle (R), after 30 years service to the hospital,
accepts transistor radio from Dr. Wadley Glenn.

JAMES TUGGLE

James Tuggle once said, "Dr. Fischer helped me out—he gave me a job. And I've stayed to help the hospital anyway I can." During James Tuggle's many years of service as head houseman, he helped train new housekeeping employees. This included his wife Eva who worked at Crawford Long for six years.

He advanced to the position of head orderly in the Operating Room where he worked until he retired after thirty-two years of service.

Mr. Tuggle died in February of 1973.

BYRON WORKERS—Venera Appling, Ruth Duncan, Minnie Simms and Willie Humphries

The Byron Apartments, a seven-story structure on Peachtree Street, were opened to full-time Crawford Long employees after they were built in 1970. Venera Appling, Resident Manager, and

Ruth Duncan, RN, made their homes at the Byron. Mrs. Appling said she especially enjoyed meeting and getting to know residents from other countries. She said, "They came from the Philippines, Korea, India, Turkey, Greece, England, and South America. One family came from China. They had such interesting stories to tell." At the time of the interview, Mrs. Appling had been working at Crawford Long for twenty-three and a half years.

Mrs. Duncan had worked thirty-eight years, including duty as head nurse on 2-B, when she moved to the Byron Apartments.

Minnie Simms, daytime housekeeper, worked at the Byron from 4 p.m. - 10 p.m. patrolling the apartment parking lot after her full day's work. She was a sixteen-year veteran worker at Crawford Long when she was featured in "The Larynx."

Today Ms. Simms and long-time Crawford Long employee, Willie Humphries, are co-resident managers of the Byron.

SUE MARTIN

In April of 1970, when Sue Martin was halfway through her twenty-fourth year at Crawford Long, she reviewed her work as an inventory clerk. In the beginning, she and a male supervisor did all the work in the storeroom. They managed the incoming items and distribution of everything from paper clips to baby formula. "Disposables have been a Godsend for the hospital and the patient," said Mrs. Martin. "Nearly everything today is either sterile, disposable or both."

EVA VAUGHN

When Eva Vaughn retired in 1971 after twenty-one years of service as a housemother to pre-graduate nursing students, she took

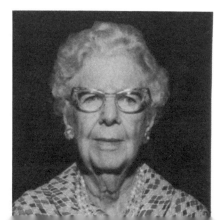

Mrs. Eva Vaughan at a reception in her honor.

memories of hundreds of hours spent with them.

The students called her "Ma" Vaughn. Many of "her girls" who went on to become nurses, wives and mothers came to her retirement party to help her celebrate.

GERALDINE OSLIN

Geraldine Oslin, chosen as the Crawford Long Employee-of-the-month in May 1971, marked thirty-three years of work in the cafeteria. She was nominated by fellow employees for extra touches that added attractiveness to the food served to patients. Her interest in food service began early in her life. Her mother, Mrs. Lillian Morris, worked in dietary.

GRACE MEADOWS

Grace Meadows, mother of twelve children including three sets of twins, was recognized in 1972 for "Her loyalty, leadership, high standards of performance, and for her sunny temperament." Mrs. Meadows had as her responsibility the coordination of the work of six other cooks in the preparation of 2,000 meals a day in the Dietary Department.

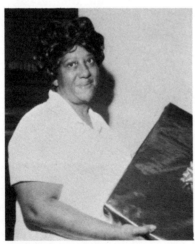
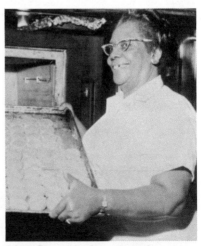

Mrs. Geraldine Oslin receives the 35-year award.

Mrs. Grace Meadows at work.

Mr. Billy Morton, Director of Environmental Services.

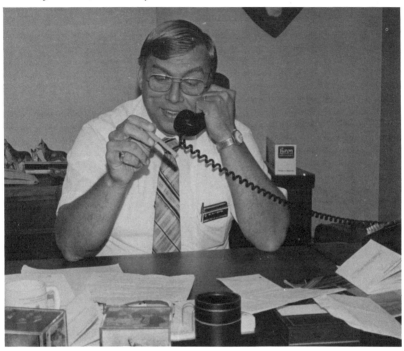

BILLY MORTON

Keeping a hospital clean and sanitary is a task that is never finished. Billy Morton, Director of Environmental Services, said of his work at Crawford Long, "I stumbled into it—it's housekeeping and I like it." He came to Crawford Long in July of 1973 after working at a nursing home and other hospitals.

He has cleaning facts and figures at his finger tips. "There are 2,500 trash cans to be emptied every day," he said. "A third of them are emptied two and three times a day. There are 10,000 light fixtures to be cleaned once a year. We have 4,000,000 square feet of wall space to be washed one or two times a year. Some of the operating rooms are washed daily. Powerful germicides with a phenol base insure sterile, germ free cleanliness.

"Housekeeping is more complex than just sweeping or mopping," Mr. Morton said. "We also clean furniture and upholstery, carpeting and the elevators. Linens are washed in 200° water and commercial grade bleaches and soap to get them both sparkling white and germ free."

"We have a crew of one hundred and thirty people, working three shifts, twenty-four hours a day, seven days a week.

"We are also responsible for pest control and the disposal of 6,000 pounds of garbage a day. Contaminated stuff is disposed by autoclave or is incinerated."

No longer do student nurses scrub floors as they did in the early days. Today twelve automatic floor scrubbers whir down corridors, cleaning as they go, scrubbing and polishing in one operation. Only clean water is put on the floor, so there's no possibility of carrying contamination from one place to the another. All floors are left dry eliminating wet, slippery floors.

"We are the image maker of the hospital," said Mr. Morton. "We go on the philosophy a clean hospital gives a good impression, sets the tone and standard for the rest of the service."

Mr. Morton has attended courses at the University of Oklahoma, and Georgia State University, and has long been active in the National Executive Housekeepers Association.

CECIL CHATHAM

Cecil Chatham came to Crawford Long Hospital as Director of Security in 1982. After a thirty-two year career with the Atlanta Police Department, he retired with rank of lieutenant. He feels his work at the hospital is more in the nature of deterring crime rather than the apprehension of criminals.

There are fifty-six employees on the security staff. All of them attend Atlanta Area Tech for security training and for pistol training on the firing range. Upon completion of the course, and after undergoing thorough FBI checks, they are issued private detective licenses by the State of Georgia. Periodically, instructors from the Georgia Police Academy give further security training and update the staff on new laws.

Since Mr. Chatham came to Crawford Long, the hospital has purchased two scooters. "I don't think we could get along without them now that the hospital is so large. The scooters have battery connections to get employees' cars started. They also carry a jack. We change tires . . . when needed," he said.

RICHARD FISHER

Richard Fisher, former Chief Therapist of the Department of Respiratory Therapy at Crawford Long Hospital was named "Delegate of the Year 1974" by the American Association for Respiratory Therapy (AART) at its national convention in Dallas, Texas.

Mr. Fisher, who served as Respiratory Therapy Advisor to Georgia State University and Emory University, was mentioned as being associated with the American Heart Association, Muscular Dystrophy Association, Public Health Association and the Pulmonary Disease Task Force of the Georgia Regional Medical Program.

CAROLYN B. HARRIS

Following her graduation from high school in 1963, Carolyn Bradley came to Crawford Long willing to undertake any task. In her twenty years of employment, she served as a personnel interviewer, a nurse recruiter, and writer and editor of the "Larynx." She also devoted herself to numerous committees and projects.

In 1983 she married Dr. Erl Harris and continues to work for the hospital part time.

CAROLYN OVERBY

Crawford Long employees often utilize their "off time" in interesting ways.

Carolyn Overby, who completed nine years of work as Personnel Assistant in April of 1974, with her husband and children was featured in the NBC News Special "White Collar America." Filmed in the Overby home and at Stone Mountain, the special was aired March 17, 1974.

Mrs. Overby also taught at the Patricia Stevens' Career College and Finishing School in Atlanta in addition to her regular duties at the hospital.

FIVE WORKERS GIVE 117 YEARS OF SERVICE

It is no secret Crawford Long employees are loyal to the hospital; many stay for years.

At one retirement party in January of 1972, five people retired with a total of one hundred and seventeen years of service.

Estelle Hilton, RN worked in Orthopedics and as head nurse on 3-B for thirty-eight years.

Anna Lee Calhoun worked in the Laundry Department for twenty-eight years.

Myrtie Steele dispensed supplies and worked with hospital printing for twenty-two years.

Martha Peterson worked for sixteen years in the Sewing Room.

Reams Latimer worked as a Dietary Department aide for thirteen years.

THREE SEAMSTRESSES

Carolyn Dunn, Estelle Kirk, and Gladys Avery spent many hours turning out doctors scrub gowns and hats, shirts and sheets, OR and OB boots, bed pan and pillow covers, swing and high chair covers as well as baby dresses and laundry bag covers.

In March of 1974, they were spotlighted for making six hundred scrub gowns in less than four months.

These industrious ladies were able to cut out and finish an OR doctor's gown in fifty-five minutes. They also mended many items that might otherwise have had to be discarded.

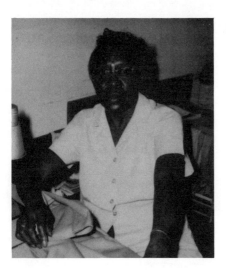

Mrs. Gladys Avery at work.

FRANCES MACKY

Frances Macky, head cook in the Dietary Department in 1974, came to work at Crawford Long Hospital in 1946 when the Woodruff Building was just being finished.

During the twenty-eight years she worked, she earned the affection of her co-workers. Kitchen crew members were lavish in praise of her in July 1974 when she was named "Employee of the Month."

Mrs. Macky was reported as saying she "thinks nothing" of preparing 2,000 meals a day.

Mrs. Macky retired in February 1987 after 41 years of service.

MICHAEL PENDER

In 1974, Michael Pender came to work at Crawford Long Hospital as a physical therapist. Praised for his sense of humor, friendliness and diligence, the Vietnam veteran followed his mother and sister, both registered nurses, into the medical field.

Mr. Pender said he came into Physical Therapy because he enjoyed working with people who needed help in rehabilitation and overcoming handicaps brought as a result of injury or illness. He felt his part was to get patients back into the mainstream of normal living again.

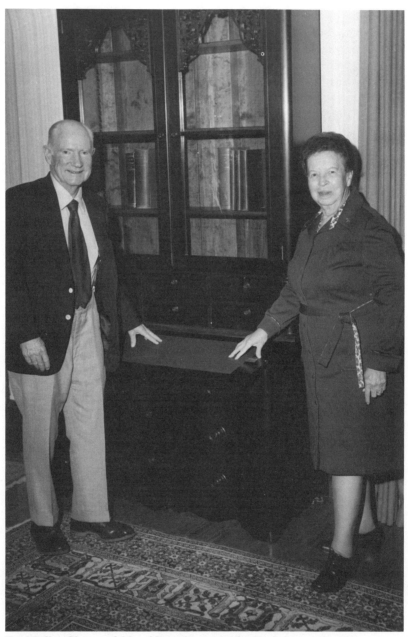

Dr. Wadley Glenn and Mrs. Nancy Yarn pose by Dr. Long's secretary.

CHAPTER SIXTEEN

THE MUSEUM

The Crawford Long Museum, located just off the lobby of the hospital in the Peachtree Tower houses books, records, medical instruments and other historical memorabilia deserving a place to be exhibited and stored for future generations. The Museum opened on Doctor's Day, March 30, 1981.

Mrs. Nancy Yarn organized the Museum and worked with Dr. Glenn to assemble, arrange and catalogue gathered materials. Impetus for the establishment of the museum came from Dr. Joe Craver, a Crawford Long Hospital staff member, and Dr. W. R. Wallace of Chester, South Carolina who realized the need for a special place dedicated to the preservation of some original Long papers given to Crawford Long Hospital by the University of South Carolina.

On display in the Museum are original early Georgia-made furniture pieces, early doctors' records hand-written in pencil in lined notebooks, Nursing School yearbooks, and histories of Crawford Long War Units. On the Museum shelves are books and copies of papers that helped establish proof that Dr. Crawford Long was indeed the first physician to use ether to induce "sleep" that would alleviate the pain of surgery.

Dr. Long's stately mahogany secretary, now beautifully restored was purchased when Mrs. Yarn learned of its existence in the J. H. Elliott Museum across the street from the hospital. The desk, dating back to 1845 owners, was purchased by Crawford Long Hospital for $3,000. The purchase price was donated by staff physicians and hospital employees. Dr. Frank K. Boland, Jr. was given a Duncan Phyfe-style table by the Long family. He in turn gave it to the museum.

Ten scrapbooks, compiled by Mrs. Yarn, preserve pictures, media reports of hospital activities and achievements, letters and thank-you notes written by grateful patients. One overflowing scrapbook tells of Dr. Fischer's work at the hospital, and about life on his farm. There is also a file of the Crawford Long in-house bulletins, the "Larynx." A portrait of Dr. Long, painted in a formal style by Winonah Bell, rests on an easel at the far end of the Museum. The Bell painting was presented to the hospital in 1935 by the Crawford Long Chapter of the United Daughters of the Confederacy. Dr. Long's daughter, Mrs. Eugenia Long Harper, then a resident of College Park, Georgia, was present for the unveiling of the portrait. Eleanore Miles, of the United Daughters of the Confederacy Children's Group, presented the picture to Dr. Fischer, who accepted it for the hospital. Another portrait, recently donated to the Museum by Dr. Long's great grandchildren, will be hung in an honored spot. This portrait, distinguished by luminous eyes that follow the viewer from any angle, was painted by one of Dr. Long's daughters. (It's not known which daughter painted the portrait.) All of the Long girls were talented artists, according to family lore.

In 1979 Dr. Stanley Peek presented Crawford Long Hospital a replica of the statue of Dr. Long in the Hall of Fame in Washington, D.C. Originally owned by Dr. Joe Jacobs (of the Atlanta Jacobs Drug Stores) the replica was sold to Hugh B. Johnson who presented it to Dr. Peek.

Dr. Crawford W. Long's name was recalled on March 30, 1987, when aportion of the observance of Doctor's Day took place in the hospital Museum. There Dr. Long's gold pocket watch was presented by his great grandchildren—Mr. Edward C. Long of Norris, Tennessee and his sister, Mrs. Frances Long Sachs of Atlanta.

Mr. Long, like his grandfather, graduated from the University of Georgia with honors for scholarly achievements. He has taught school and worked at Oak Ridge as a technical supervisor in Calutron Uranium isotopes separation at the Tennessee Eastman Corporation.

Mrs. Sachs also inherited the Long family love of scientific study. She graduated from Vanderbilt with a degree in civil engineering, at a time when women were limited to school teaching or music instruction if they wished to work. She also attended the University of Georgia, the University of Tennessee, William and Mary College, and the University of Maryland. She said, with a grin, "I'm a perpetual student." She worked at Oak Ridge as a nuclear engineer.

The Crawford Long Museum guest book, started in Novem-

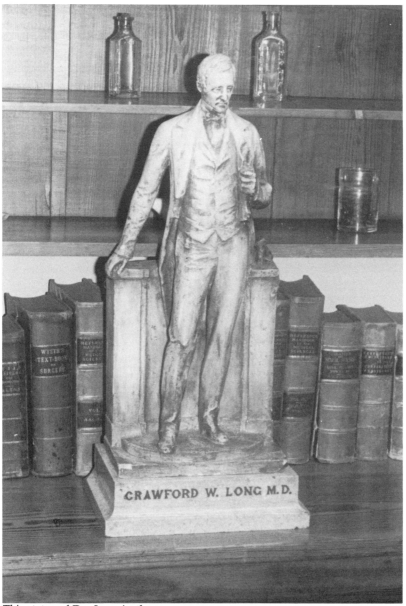

This statue of Dr. Long in the
hospital museum is a replica
of the one that stands in Washington, D.C.

ber 1983, has been signed by people from all over the United States.

Other Museum volunteers are Alice Martin, RN, Elizabeth Koppe, and RosAnne Jones. They act as guides to visitors, adult and school children groups, patients and staff members.

Patsy Wiggins, appointed Museum Coordinator in November 1985, has brought to the position professional experience gained in her work at the Atlanta Historical Society and the DeKalb Historical Society. She is responsible for acquisitions and care of the Museum artifacts.

EXHIBITS OF INTEREST

Medical instruments, an early patient "feeding bowl," a field lamp used during the War Between the States, and medicine bottles.

Dr. Davis' Spanish American and World War I uniforms.

A Crawford Long nurse's uniform and cap.

A replica of the 1865 pardon by President Johnson freeing Dr. Long to treat United States Army troops stationed in North Georgia.

A letter from Dr. E. G. Ballenger to Eugenia Long Harper.

A signed copy of "Some Personal Recollections and Private Correspondence of Dr. Crawford Williamson Long"—Jos. Jacobs PHAR, Atlanta, Ga. 1919.

A letter to Mrs. Long from Dr. Long dated April 26, 1854.

Copy of a breezy column by the late Billy Rose praising doctors.

Sets of early medical books, a telephone from the 1908 era and many other items of interest to history lovers.

A DREAM FOR THE FUTURE

Back in 1964, Dr. John M. Brown, Dick Fisher, and Laura Blackwell had a dream of founding a Museum of Respiratory Science at Crawford Long. This future museum would be known as the Museum of Respiratory Science, and would contain photographs, biographical sketches and taped interviews with living pioneers of respiratory therapy. Dr. Brown was one of those pioneers.

In 1973, respiratory therapists at Crawford Long started a collection of items that played a significant role in the development of respiratory science.

Dr. Glenn designated a temporary storage place for the collection of artifacts in the Prescott Street Building.

With the decline of polio, once the major crippler and killer of children in the United States, many devices developed during that period have become obsolete. As the field of respiratory science modernized, many devices became objects of historical interest only.

Laura Blackwell, of the Crawford Long Respiratory Therapy Department, said there was a large response from all across the nation commending the effort to save the material.

Dr. John M. Brown, Chief of Anesthesiology at Crawford Long at the time said, "Many pioneers in respiratory science are still living. But we feel that without a museum, a suitable place for collection, display and preservation of artifacts and historical data to preserve them, they will be lost."

Dr. Brown arranged to pick up antiquated equipment in various cities in three trips because he believed the pieces too valuable to be shipped. Some items are the original works of Joseph Priestly, the discoverer of oxygen.

Bill Moore, Chief Engineer, has refurbished an iron lung which was exhibited during Hospital Week at Crawford Long in 1987.

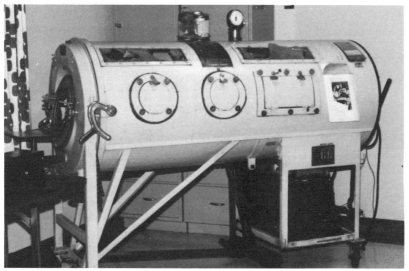

The refurbished iron lung.

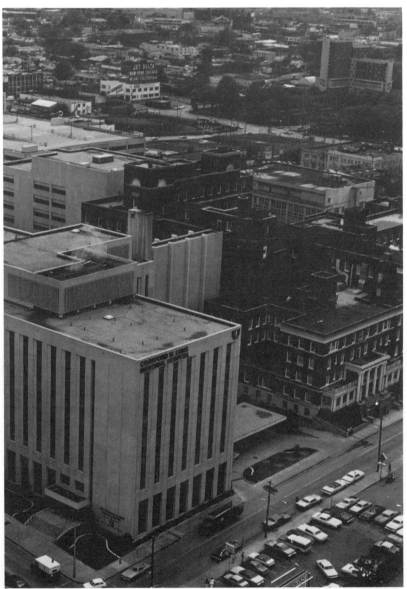

Crawford Long Hospital

SUMMING UP

Many years have passed since Dr. E. C. Davis and Dr. L. C. Fischer began their small sanitarium in 1908. Family names prominent in Atlanta and Georgia's history are interwoven with the recorded advancement of Crawford Long's goal to be an institution for all people as envisioned by its pioneer founders.

Graduates of the Crawford Long School of Nursing, one thousand, eight hundred and forty-six in number, have left their imprint on the hospital.

Many of the early graduates still meet to keep alive the ties forged when nurses' training included many tasks no longer required of students.

Martha Huey, an early graduate, spoke of semi-annual get togethers the Alumnae Group have at Christmas time and a picnic in July. "Then we have a covered dish lunch and have the best time talking. We are so happy to be together. We are just family."

Mrs. Huey was a member of the first class of eleven girls graduating under the name of Crawford Long Hospital in 1934. She has been the Alumnae treasurer for twelve years and retains enthusiasm for the long friendships the members have retained since their student days. All fifty members, including one who sends her dues from Michigan, keep in touch with each other.

Mrs. Lillian Hutchinson Miller, a 1939 Crawford Long graduate, recently stopped off at Crawford Long while en route to her home in Florida with her husband, Dr. Charles Miller, to show him her "old stomping ground." Now retired from thirty years of nursing, she well remembers her student days. She said, "We rushed with so much to do, with so many wards, maybe four or five, with patients to bathe, medicate and so forth before 9 o'clock. Students today don't do that. I feel the change is for the better. But I liked it here, working with Dr. Frank Kells Boland and his son. It was a busy time but I enjoyed it.

"We wore, as students, a long blue uniform, a white apron, white hose and shoes. Now things have changed, even since I retired in 1978 as a V.A. nurse. Everything is computerized now."

Mrs. Reba Trean, now principal at the Sylvan Hills Elementary School in Atlanta, remembers her work as a medical secretary for Dr. Frank Kells Boland, Jr. after World War II.

She said she once asked him why he worked so hard, sometimes twenty hours a day. She shook her head as she said he told her that when he was in the thick of battle, he made a vow that if he ever got home, he would never turn a patient away, no matter the hour of the day or the person's financial status.

"And he didn't," she added. "His son, Frank III, was the first Crawford Long baby to have a complete blood transfusion. The nurses loved Dr. Boland because he always had a smile for them and a little trinket he gave to everyone he met. You never knew what he might hand out—rain bonnets in little boxes, sewing kits or lipsticks."

When the mayor of a Michigan city came to Atlanta for a convention in 1970, he had no idea of spending Christmas there or that his wife would be a patient in Crawford Long Hospital far away from home and family. However, when his wife suffered a gallbladder attack that demanded emergency surgery and a long convalescence, he commuted between Atlanta and Michigan. With his time so divided between duty and family obligations, he expected to spend Christmas away from his wife.

Then he changed his mind, he said, "Because everyone down here had been so nice and thoughtful to me and my wife, I decided to bring my two kids down here for Christmas in Crawford Long Hospital."

A trimmed tree, presents under it in the sick woman's room, led the man to say, "The best present our whole family got was a warm reception by you Southerners and the great therapeutic help my wife got by your friendliness. All the hospital people did everything they could possibly do to make us feel at home . . . When I get back home, I will carry with me the spirit of Christmas I found here in Atlanta." His wife said, "You people down here really have it."

A letter to the hospital in 1980 began, "you're No. 1." It went on to say, "My wife and I probably have logged more days, as patients, in Crawford Long than many of your regular employees.

"I was born and lived the first two weeks of my life in an incubator on the second floor of the 'old' building. That was in 1924. My younger brother and sister were both born at Crawford Long.

Thirty-three years ago on December 7, 1946, our daughter made her appearance at the same time the emergency rooms and adjacent corridors were filled with victims of the tragic Winecoff fire which claimed 112 lives.

"Two years later, our son arrived. Where else?—the Maternity Ward in the 'old' building.

"Since then the two of us have occupied almost every floor in both the old and new wings. We have always been blessed with competent, courteous and compassionate service from most of the staff, but this is to tell you during the past two weeks in Wing 6100, each and every one of you won the title No. 1 in our book. Best wishes for a Happy Holiday season."

Another patient gives credit to a seventeen minute helicopter trip that brought him to the Crawford Long Emergency room and successful treatment. It began when a man, stricken on a Fayetteville Street, was taken to his doctor's office where an electrocardiogram showed he was experiencing a heart attack. The helicopter was summoned and he was brought to Crawford Long where help waited.

Doctor Douglas Morris, Cardiologist, and a team of nurses injected a new drug into the patient's arm to dissolve a blood clot stopping up one of the man's coronary arteries.

An anxious mother from Mississippi flew into Atlanta in the fall of 1986 to the bedside of her daughter who became an emergency patient at Crawford Long when she was suddenly struck with appendicitis.

"I'm so relieved my daughter is alright," she said. "I can't get over the fact she became ill while on her way to the football game in Athens, and was brought by a stranger to the Crawford Long Emergency Clinic where she was treated so promptly. The Business Office people were so kind. They called us but the hospital had already started treatment for her even as we were giving insurance information over the phone. I will always appreciate this care for my daughter and the kindness of the people I have met here."

THE SPIRIT OF CRAWFORD LONG

In January of 1982, Dr. Glenn showed his gratitude in a letter directed to all hospital personnel to thank them for their support during a snow storm.

Dr. Glenn wrote: "We have always prided ourselves on having a close knit hospital family that cares. The teamwork that was so prevalent throughout the weather of January 12-16, 1982, was most outstanding.

"Our employees willingly worked long hours to see that our patients were given the best care possible under extremely adverse conditions. Many employees volunteered to sleep at the hospital to insure that they would be at the hospital for their shift.

"Mrs. Ann Stroud and her staff kept the School of Nursing dormitory open for hospital staff to be bedded down. Student nurses and School of Nursing faculty supplemented the nursing staff on patient units.

"Mrs. Georgia Belle Martin and the Byron Apartment staff utilized vacant apartments to house employees during the storm. The Dietary Department kept the cafeteria open longer hours to insure that medical staff, employees and visitors would have an opportunity to be served food.

"Employees with four-wheel drive vehicles volunteered to pick up other employees. Ancillary support services performed in an outstanding manner.

"Miss Katherine Pope and her nursing staff not only took care of our patients but also made sure that visitors, physicians and employees were housed.

New help in Dietary during the snow storm
included Sid Swilley from Engineering and Mary Walton
and Barbara White from Personnel.

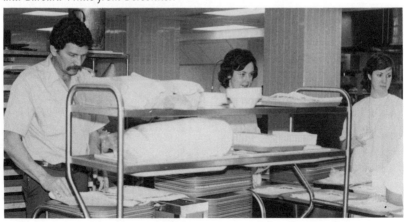

"Patients did not miss a single meal being served on time. This was possible because the dietary tray assembly line was supplemented by employees from the Personnel Department, Materials Management and Engineering. Mr. Robert M. Kimble, Mr. P. Douglas Bennett and Mr. Render S. Davis worked on the tray line also. This type of teamwork exemplifies the attitudes that most of our employees demonstrated during the storm.

"Mr. John D. Henry reported that he received many compliments from patients and their families for care rendered. Mr. Henry also visited with patients on each nursing unit. Patients were most appreciative of the care rendered them under these severe weather conditions. We are confident that we will receive more compliments for your outstanding performance.

"Mr. Barker, Mr. Henry, Mr. Davis and I thank you for a job well done and we are mighty proud of each of you."

CRAWFORD LONG HOSPITAL
AUXILIARY ROSTER
MAY 1987

Mrs. Loura Aiken
Mrs. Mary Almon
Mrs. Thomas J. Anderson, Jr.
Ms. Carolyn Anglin
Mrs. Cleo Arnold
Mrs. Jeff Bachman
Mrs. Robert J. Bachman
Mrs. W. Daniel Barker
Mrs. Louis Battey
Mrs. Frank Bedinger
Mrs. Linton H. Bishop
Mrs. Albert Blackwelder
Mrs. Jack Bleich
Mrs. Virginia Mae Blum
Mrs. Max M. Blumberg
Mrs. Walter W. Bolton III
Mrs. William Bondurant
Mrs. John Bostwick
Mrs. Henry Bourne
Mrs. Stephen Bowles
Mrs. O. M. Bradford
Miss Betty Braver
Mrs. Glenn Bridges, Jr.
Mrs. Morris Brown
Mrs. Nelson Brown
Mrs. Gary Howard Burgess
Mrs. Mary Jane Burns
Mrs. Rebecca Caccavale
Mrs. Grace Caldwell
Mrs. F. Phinizy Calhoun, Jr.
Mrs. Andrew Carlos
Mr. George Castleberry
Mrs. Donald C. Chait
Miss Frances Clark
Miss Julia Clements
Mrs. J. Luther Clements
Mrs. John D. Clendenen
Mrs. John H. Clifton
Mrs. Jewell Cofer
Mrs. John Coleman
Mrs. Sara G. Cone
Mrs. Mary Cook
Mrs. William Crowe
Mrs. Margaret Daniel

Mrs. Rubye David
Mrs. Guy Davis
Mrs. Render S. Davis
Mrs. William Davis
Mrs. Paul W. DeFoor
Mrs. Jacinto del Mazo
Mrs. Clifton Dillman
Mrs. James Dodds
Mrs. Earl Dolive
Mrs. James Dolive
Miss Lynne Dorsey
Mrs. James Duke
Mrs. Walter S. Dunbar
Ms. Peggy Dunn
Mrs. George Dyer
Mrs. Elizabeth Easterling
Mrs. Boone Ellis
Mrs. Jack H. Elrod
Mrs. E. A. Feliciano
Mrs. Sara Field
Ms. Dorothy Fierst
Mrs. George J. Fleeman
Mr. & Mrs. Stanley Floersheim
Mrs. J. Gilbert Foster
Mrs. Eric Frankel
Mrs. Isobel Fraser
Mrs. Edna L. Fritschel
Mrs. Sylvia Galanti
Mrs. Franklin M. Garrett
Mrs. Dorothy Gilner
Mrs. Frances L. Glenn
Mrs. Thomas K. Glenn II
Mrs. W. Kearney Glenn
Mrs. Claude Grizzard, Jr.
Mrs. Gilbert D. Grossman
Mrs. Morton Gruber
Mrs. Mary Will Guest
Mrs. Robert Guyton
Mrs. L. Harvey Hamff
Miss Gladys Hancock
Mrs. Robert Ken Hancock
Mrs. Daniel D. Hankey
Mrs. William C. Hatcher
Mrs. Gene Hauck

Mrs. John D. Henry
Mrs. Robert T. Henson
Mrs. Mary Helen Herndon
Mrs. James J. Hicks
Miss Nelda Hill
Mrs. Luther C. Hitchcock
Mrs. Charles Holloway
Mrs. Petie Holloway
Mrs. Donald Hooper
Mrs. Ruth Hudgins
Mrs. Ellis R. Jackson
Mrs. Mack A. Jones
Mrs. Elijah Jordan
Mrs. Ralph Keith
Mrs. Daniel Kingloff
Mrs. Jacob I. Kingloff
Miss Mary Aline Kinsey
Mrs. Grace Kirk
Miss Elizabeth A. Koppe
Mrs. Paul A. Lavietes
Mrs. Raye Levinson
Mrs. Henry Liberman
Mrs. Dan Lockman
Mrs. R. Bruce Logue
Mrs. Julian Lokey
Mrs. Wilton Looney
Mrs. Edwin Macon
Mrs. Allen Macris
Mrs. James Magbee
Mrs. Kamal Mansour
Mrs. Betty Marcus
Mrs. Alice Martin
Ms. Del Martin
Mrs. Vesta Masters
Mrs. Joseph Mayson
Mrs. Spence McClelland
Mrs. John McCraney
Mrs. William McKinnon
Mrs. Margaret Meals
Mrs. Ruth E. Mendenhall
Mrs. Helen H. Merriam
Mrs. Ivan Miles
Mrs. Robert Milledge
Mrs. Joseph Miller

Mrs. William W. Moore, Jr.
Mrs. J. W. Morgan
Mrs. Douglas C. Morris
Mrs. Steven J. Morris
Mrs. Roy G. Moss
Mrs. Eva Nabors
Mrs. Foad Nahai
Mrs. Edmund Nicholas
Mrs. Merv W. Nickel
Mrs. John E. Nickerson
Mrs. Carol Olley
Mrs. Hernando T. Ortega
Mrs. Francis Owings
Mrs. T. Harding Paine
Mrs. Bernard H. Palay
Mrs. Randolph Patterson
Mrs. William J. Pendergrast, Sr.
Mrs. W. Jefferson Pendergrast, Jr.
Mrs. Matilda Pinhas
Mrs. J. E. Plunkett
Mrs. Marion Pool
Mrs. Audrey Poulos
Mrs. Viva Powell

Mrs. Mary Catherine Ramos
Mrs. Fran Rankine
Mrs. A. Cullen Richardson
Mrs. Frances Inez Rikard
Mrs. David L. Roos, Jr.
Mrs. Frank Rumph
Mrs. Virginia Sammons
Mrs. Clarence N. Scheinbaum
Miss Rubye Seay
Mrs. Warren P. Sewell
Mrs. Joseph Sierer
Mrs. George M. Skardasis
Mrs. Charles W. Smith
Mrs. Robert R. Snodgrass
Mrs. Jerry Staton
Mrs. Collier St. Clair
Mrs. Saul D. Stein
Mrs. Thomas Stelson
Mrs. Ron Stephens
Mrs. Marguerite Stillerman
Mrs. Bernard Ray Sturm
Mrs. Julian Swann
Mrs. Gregory S. Thompson

Mrs. Roy S. Thompson, Jr.
Mrs. William E. Thorneloe
Mrs. Bryan H. Timberlake
Mrs. Dennis Turner, Jr.
Miss Mary Turner
Mrs. Marion Vardaman
Mrs. Jesse W. Veatch, Jr.
Ms. Geneva Verdery
Mrs. Thomas Vietch
Mrs. Cosetta Walker
Mrs. G. Edward Walker
Mrs. Rachel Watson
Mrs. Carolyn Webb
Mrs. Ben L. Weinberg
Mrs. Irving W. Whiteman
Miss Patsy A. Wiggins
Mrs. Merle B. Wildman
Mrs. Walter Wildstein
Mrs. Jimmie Williams
Mrs. Joseph Wilson
Mrs. Louis A. Wilson
Mrs. James H. Wood
Mrs. Ben H. Zimmerman

PAST AUXILIARY PRESIDENTS
(Honorary Members)

1954-1956	Mrs. J. Luther Clements	1969-1971	Mrs. Robert T. Henson
1956-1957	*Mrs. Grace Archbold	1971-1973	*Mrs. C. Stedman Glisson
1957-1958	Mrs. Geneva (Mac) Verdery	1973-1975	*Mrs. R. Rollison
1958-1959	Mrs. Eva Nabors	1975-1977	Mrs. Robert T. Henson
1959-1961	*Mrs. R. A. Elmer	1977-1979	Mrs. T. Harding Paine
1961-1962	Mrs. A. Cullen Richardson	1979-1981	Mrs. George Dyer
1961-1964	Mrs. Jack H. Elrod	1981-1983	Mrs. Clarence N. Scheinbaum
1964-1965	*Mrs. J. Q. Maxwell	1983-1985	Mrs. J. Gilbert Foster, Jr.
1965-1967	Mrs. Ruth E. Mendenhall	1985-1986	*Mrs. Joseph Mayson
1967-1969	Mrs. Marguerite Stillerman	1986-1987	Mrs. Donald C. Chait

* Deceased

INDEX

Numbers in **bold** refer to pictures or illustrations.

Abbott, Jack, 159, 162, **162**
Acklin, A. A., 16, **16**
Adams, Pat, 38
Administration, 153-169
Air Conditioning, 95-96
Alexander, King of Greece, 6
Allen Triplets, 96, **96**
Almada, E. L., 15
Anderson, Margaret, **183**
Anesthesiology Department, 150
Anglin, Carolyn, 146, **164**, 167
Appling, Venera, 188
Auxiliary to the Crawford Long
  Hospital, 113, 121-133
  Members of the Auxiliary (1987), 208
Aven, Carl C., 17
Avery, Gladys, 194, **194**
Babin, Ruth, 36-37, **73**
Bachman, Robert J., 168
Ballenger, Edgar G., 6
Barfield, F. M., 6
Barfield, Otis, 126
Barker, W. Daniel, 15, 107, **116**, 135, **152**, 153-157, **178**, **186**, 207
Barnett, Gladys Smith, **32**
Base Hospital No. 43, 71
  Nurses of Base Hospital No. 43, **70**
Bennett, P. Douglas, **154**, 207
Bishop, Linton H. Jr., 131, 137
Blackwell, Laura, 200
Block, Bates, 3
Boland, Frank Kells, 6, 16, 23-24, **23**, 31, **69**, 72
Boland, Frank Kells Jr., **73**, 76-78, 197, 204
Boland, Joseph H., 17, 73
Bolton, Frances Payne, 45
Bouknight, Mendal, 166, **166**
Bradley, Carolyn, 124
Bradley, W. H., **98**
Braude, James, **107**, 107-108
Brockman, Mary, **25**
Broughton, Len G., 3

Brown, John M., 200
Brundage, Anna, 34
Bunce, Allen H., 6
Bunce, Isabella Arnold, 4-5
Burt, George R., 15
Cadet Nurse Training Program, 44-49, **46-47**, 82
Calhoun, Anna Lee, 194
Campbell, J. L., 17
Camp Gordon, 67
Camp Hospital No. 25, 68
Camp Livingston, 74
  Medical, Dental and Administrative
  Officers at Camp Livingston, 1942, **77**
Candler, C. H. Jr., 10
Candlish, Jessie M., 15
Carlton, H. H., 30
Carlyle Fraser Heart Center, 129-133
Carmichael, Edna, **35**
Carter, Jimmy, 42, 107
Cassels, Christine, **186**
Chapel Program, 113-119
Chappel, Amey, 19
Chatham, Cecil, 192
Chemotherapy Department, 149-150
Christian, Floye, **35**
Christian, Mozelle, **35**
Cierney, George III, 108
Civil War, 29, 33
Clements, Margaret, 122
Collins, Edna, **35**
Conklin, Robin, **127**
Cooking With Love, 124
Craver, Joe, 197
Crawford Long Museum, 197-201, **199**
Crawford W. Long Memorial Museum, 31
Crittenton, Florence, 41
Crook, Gregory, **154**, 163
Curtis, Louise, **35**
Dailey, Betty, **125**, **186**
Dalton, Margaret, **25**
Dantzler, Caroline, 70
David, Rubye, 111, 181-182
Davidson, Owen, 162
Davis, Edward Campbell, 1-21, **2**, 24, 34, 36, **66**, 67-68, 72-73, 113, 203
Davis, Eila Catherine Windler, 1
Davis, Maria Carter, 3, 4
Davis, Render S., 8, **152**, **154**, 155, 207

Davis, Robert Carter, 8
Davis, Robert Carter Jr., 8, **109**, 109-111
Davis, Shelley Carter, 2, 3, 6, **7**, 8, 38
Davis, Mrs. Shelley Carter, 4
Davis, William Lewis Gardner Davis, 1-2
Davis-Fischer Sanatorium, 1-21
Dawkins, Louise, 182
Dawson, W. C., 28
Denmark, Lola, 19
DeSmidt, Marguerite, 159
Doremus, Estes, 15
Douglas, Loyce, **74**
Dowman, Charles, 6, 97
Dozier, Albert, 72
Duckworth, Ruth, **145**
Dulaney, Virginia, **121**
Duncan, Ruth, 179, **179**, 189
Dunn, Carolyn, 194
Easterly, Mrs. J. F. Jr., **125**
Edwards, Ann, 162
Elkin, D. C., 19
Elmer, Laverne 125
Elrod, Mrs. J. H. Jr., **120**
Emergency Department, 138-139
Emily Winship Woodruff Maternity
    Center, 85-87, **86**
Emory Unit No. 43, 7, 67-73
Engineering Department, 140-142
Environmental Health Deparment, 104
Equen, Murdock, 6, 111
Ether, 27
Eubanks, Marlene, 160
Evans, Albert L., 174
Ferguson, Ira A., **74**
First Steps, 144-145
Fischer, Hartford, 10
Fischer, Lucy Hurt, 11, **11**, 14, 15
Fischer, Luther C., 1-21, **10**, **13**, **20**, 24,
    36, 51, 86, 113, 122, 158, 198, 203
Fischer, Sally Rainey, 10
Fisher, Dick, 200
Fisher, Richard, 193
Fisk, E. F. C., 82, **82**
Fitts, John, 6
Flournoy, Gil, **154**, 159, 161-162, **162**
Flowerland, 13, 14, 17
43rd General Hospital World War II-The
    Emory Unit, The, 73
Fowler, Margaret, 181

Fraser, Carlyle, **128**, 129
Fraser, Mrs. Carlyle, 129, **130**
French, Daniel, 92
Garrett, Franklin, 11
Garson, Greer, 87-88
Gastrointestinal Laser Endoscopy, 109-111
Giddens, Donald, 144
Gift for Life, 136-137
Glenn, Agnes Raoul, 52
Glenn, Evelyn McCoy, **58**
Glenn, Frances Lewis, 52-54, **60**
Glenn, Thomas K., 16, **16**, 52, 63
Glenn, Wadley Raoul, 16, **16**, 38, 51-65,
    54, **55**, **57**, **60**, **64**, 79, **116**, **120**, 129, **140**,
    152, **188**, **196**, 197, 205-207
Glenn, Wadley Raoul, Jr., 53
Glenn, Rev. Wilbur F., 52
Glenn, Wilbur F., 17, **61**, 61
Glenn, William Kearney, 53, **60**
Glenn Building, 137
Glisson, Fred L., 116
Grant, George R., 26
Great Depression, 36
Greene, Edgar H., 6
Greene, Edward H., 17
Greenhill, James, 166-167
Greer, Molly, **back cover**
Grossman, Gilbert, 132
Gruentzig, Andreas, 131-132, **133**
Guyton, Robert, 144
Hampton, Patrick N. B., 73
Hancock, Thomas H., 15
Harper, Eugenia Long, 24, **25**
Harriman, Jane, 160
Harris, Carolyn B., 193
Harris, Joe Frank Jr., 102
Harrison, Ruth, **35**
Hart, Mary G., **184**, 185
Hatcher, Charles R. Jr., 63, 131
Hatcher, Margaret Brown Nursing
    Education Center, 139-140
Hatcher, Peggy **140**
Hatcher, William, **130**, 140, **140**
Hayes, James A., 52
Haynes, C. Doyle, 174-175, **175**
Henderson, Bessie, **76**
Henry, John, **127**, **152**, 157-158, **179**, 207
Henson, Mrs. Robert "Coc", 24, 126-127,
    127

Hilton, Estelle, 194
History of the Emory Base Unit No. 43,
  67, 70
Hoke, Michael, 3
Holmes, J. B. S., 2-3
Hooker, Ina, 105
Horsley, Joyce, **183**
Hubbard, Mamie Lowe, 92
Huckaby, Louis F., **112**, 114, **116**
Huey, Martha, 203
Humphries, Willie, 189
Hurst, Lura, **35**
Hurt, Charles Davis III, 14
Hurt, Charles D., 3, 11, 14
Hurt, Joel, 14
Hurt, Melissa Jack, 14
Hyde, Sara, 115
Iron Lung, **201**
Jacobs, Joseph, 24, 27, 198
Jackson, Charles, 28
Jackson, Leroy, **back cover**
Jackson, Maynard, 60
Jenkins, Frank, 117
Jenkins, Mattie Jean, 182
Jenkins, Ralph, 182
Johnson, Glenice, **back cover**
Johnson, Martha, **40**
Jones, Boisfeuillet, 10
Jones, Harold D., 117, **119**
Jones, Tom, 79
Joselyn, Lillian, 34
Kimble, Robert M., **154**, 207
King, Dudley, 172
Kirk, Estelle, 194
LaFrage, Susan W., **74**
Lambie, Jeanne, 37
Lane, Evangeline, 38
Latimer, Reams, 194
Laundry Department, 136
Lawrence, Charles E., 6
Leach, Willaford Ransom, 139
Leach, Anna Winship, 139
Lee, Betty, 91
Lee, Mary, 35
"Lethon", 27
Lifeline, 145-146
Logue, R. Bruce, 130
Long, Mary Caroline Swain, 28, 30
Long, Crawford Williamson, 22-31, **22**,
  33, 197-198

Long, Edward C., 198
Long, Emma, 24
Looney, Wilton, **131**, 131
Lorenz, Janet, 91
Lowry, Robert, 4, 12
Mabon, Robert, 75
Macky, Frances, 195
Mahoney, Clara, 182
Martin, Alice, 15, 177-178, **178**
Martin, Georgia Belle Hearn, 37, 97-98,
  176-177, **176**, 206
Martin, Shirley, **176**
Martin, Sue, 189
Massey, Joseph T. Jr., 163-164, **164**
Mattingly, Mack, 102
May, Armand, 16, **16**
Mayson, Frances Glenn, 53, **60**
McArthur, Louise, **35**
McCauley, Mrs. George R., 121
McGinley, Agnes, 34
Meadows, Grace, 190, **190**
Medical Transcription Department, 168
Meshgraft Dermatome, 99-100
Miles, Eleanor, **25**
Miller, Lillian Hutchinson, 203
Miller, Lou, 34
Miriani, Miss, **37**
Mizell, LaRue, **121**
Moffet, Ethel, **35**
Moore, William, 79, 141, **141**, 201
Morgan, Cheryl, **107**
Morgan, Edna, **37**
Morris, Douglas, 205
Morton, Billy, 191, **191**
Morton, W. T., 27, 28
Moss, Freda, 92, **92**, 165
Murray, Sara, **35**
Museum of Respiratory Science, 200-201
Newton, Gaynelle, 114
Nightingale Florence, 34
Nix, Dorothy, 87
Nuclear Medicine Department, 182-183
Olley, Mrs. J. F., **125**
Open Heart Surgery, 106
Oppenheimer, P. H., 15, 17
Oslin, Geraldine, 190, **190**
Pacer Award, 155
Peachtree Road Race, 139
Pender, Michael, 195
Pendleton, J. D., 4

Pershing, John J., 6, 9, 72
Persons, Minnie O., **74**
Peterson, Martha, 194
Poore, Jewell, **35**
Pope, Katherine, 39-44, **40**, 98, 183-184, **183**, 206
Premaure Nursery, 83-84, 104-105
Priestly, Joseph, 201
Quadruplets, **103**
Quillian, Sara, 104
Radiation Center, 137-138
Ramos, Harold, 138, **170**, 171-172
Reagan, Ronald, 102
Recovery Room, 97
Reisman, J. N., 16, **16**
Reisweber, Mary, 180
Reeves, Elsie, 180-181
Renfroe, Agnes, **73**
Reynolds, Juanita, **149**
Reynolds, Wesley, **149**
Rh Transfusion, 99
Richardson, A. C., 102
Rivers, E. D., 15
Roberts, Ada, 159-161
Roberts, Agnes, 9
Roberts, M. H., 19
Robinson, Glendora, 39, 179
Robinson, J. D., 16, **16**
Rogers, Cathy, **147**
Rollison, Mary, **125**
Roosevelt, Eleanor, 18
Rubin, Nadine, 180
Sachs, Frances Long, 198
Sanders, May, 37
Sanford, J. E., 16, **16**
Sauls, Jake, 6
School of Nursing, 36-49
Scroggins, Grace, **35**
Seigler, Helon Burton, 44-49, **44**
Sessions, Emily, 118, **119**
Shanks, Zola Lacretia Thomas, 76, **76**
Sharp, Harvey, **147**
Sheafe, Ruth, 91
Short, Sibyl, **125**, 167
Simms, Minnie, 189
Smith, Carl, 150-151
Smith, Lois, 161
Smith, Mary, 76
Social Service Department, 150
Soper, LeRoy D., **74**

Spackman, Elwood H., **118**
Spackman, Julie, 117, **118**
Steele, Myrtie, 194
Stephens, J. Ronald, 173, **173**
Stephens, Macie, 37-38, **37**, 122, 184
Stillerman, H. B., 104
Stillerman, Marguerite, 104
Strickland, W. W. Jr., 73
Strickler, Cyrus W., 6, 73
Stroud, Ann, 39, 206
Sutton, Caroline, 35
Swilley, Sid, **206**
Sylvester, Kathryn, **35**
Tanner, James C. Jr., **98**, 99-100
Tanner-Vandeput Prize, 100
Tallent, Thelma, **35**
Taylor, Frances Long, 28, 29
Taylor, Marion Smith, 82-84, **83**, 105, **149**
Temples, Mona, 124, **125**, 157
Thompson, Alice, 13, 15, **20**, 36, **49**, **94**, 95
Titus, Mrs. Richard, **121**
Trean, Reba, 204
Trial 33, 136
Tuggle, James, 188, **188**
Turman, Pollard, 137
Vandeput, Jacque, 100
Van Landingham, Michael, 159
Vaughan, Eulalia, **25**
Vaughan, Eva, 189, **189**
Veatch, Jesse W., 174
Venable, James, 27
Video Instruction, 95
Vijay, Girija, 164-165, **165**
Wadley R. Glenn Operating Pavilion, 143
Wadley R. Glenn Chair in Surgery at Emory University, 63
Walker, Dorothy, 19
Wallace, W. R., 197
Walsh, Ruth, **123**
Walton, Mary, **206**
Ward, Harriet, 180
Wardlaw, William C. Jr., 92
Wardley, Katresa, **149**
Warner, Ward, **142**
Watson, Jean, 181
Weaver, J. Calvin, 8
Wells, Horace, 28
White, Barbara, **206**
White, Goodrich C., 10
Wiggins, Patsy, 200

Williams, Cora Best Taylor, **88**, 89-90
Williams, G. A., 19
Williams, George A., 175-176
Williams, Jesse Parker, **88**, 89
Williams, Jesse Parker Hospital, **91**, 89-93
   Trustees Jesse Parker Williams Hospital
   (May 27, 1987), 93
Wilson, Woodrow, 6, 67
Winn, Jim, **116**, 117
Woo, Robert Ken Jr., 100, 101
Wood, R. H., 19

Wood, R. Hugh, **74**
Woodruff Health Sciences Center, **94**
Woodruff, Ernest, 16, **16**
Woodruff, George W., 10, 16, **16**
Woodruff, Robert, 61
Woodruff, Mrs. Robert, 121, **121**
Woolford, Guy, 16, **16**
World War I, 6, 34, 67-73
World War II, 73-79, 82
Yarn, Lisa, **back cover**
Yarn, Nancy, 124, **125**, 158-160, **196**, 197